D1737947

Inspiring Memoir

NICU MIRACLE

— BABY ZOYA —

BY LACEY M. ROBINSON

NICU Miracle:

Inspiring Memoir – Baby Zoya

This is a work of nonfiction. Events and conversations have been portrayed to the best of the author's recollection. Some names and identifying details have been changed to protect the privacy of individuals.

ISBN: 9798307765623

Imprint: Independently published

Printed in the United States of America

First Edition, 2025

DEDICATION

To my precious daughter, Zoya,
You are the light of my life and my greatest miracle.
Your courage and resilience inspire me every single day.

And to my husband, Trevor,
Your unwavering love and strength have been my anchor.
Together, we've faced every challenge and celebrated
every triumph.

This book is for you both—
My family, my heart, my everything.

ACKNOWLEDGMENTS

Abby Peto
Brittany Dreher
Caroline English
Kayla Kohler

You healed and protected our daughter with unmatched care and love, but you also became part of our family. Your unwavering support carried us through the darkest days. Your strength gave us courage, your kindness brought us comfort, and your belief in Zoya gave us hope. You will forever hold a special place in our hearts.

To the entire team of neonatologists, registered nurses, and nurse practitioners, your tireless dedication and compassion made all the difference in Zoya's journey.

To our family and friends who prayed, supported, and believed in miracles, your love lifted us and reminded us that we were never alone.

PREFACE

From the moment I knew I was going to be a mother, I dreamed of the day I would bring my baby home. This dream shaped every part of me, a promise to the life I had yet to meet. Nothing could have prepared me for the journey my family and I would face when my daughter Zoya arrived too soon, fighting for every breath in the NICU.

This book is a reflection of our story, a journey of hope, love, and resilience. It is a testament to the power of advocacy, the strength found in the most trying moments, and the miracles that unfold even in the darkest times. As I recount the highs and lows, I hope this story brings comfort to parents, inspires those walking a similar path, and shines a light on the strength within each of us to overcome.

Zoya's journey is not just about survival, it is about love, courage, and the unwavering belief in a brighter tomorrow.

— Lacey M. Robinson

TOGETHER

I have always seen myself as a traditional girl, dreaming of the day I finally meet my prince charming. The man who will sweep me off my feet, love me for who I am, and most importantly, bless me with a beautiful family of our own. For as long as I can remember, I've dreamed of a love as deep and true as the love I saw in my family. Growing up, I was surrounded by the unwavering commitment of my parents and grandparents. My parents, together since they were fifteen, have built a life rooted in love that has lasted over thirty-five years. Both sets of my grandparents have celebrated over sixty years of marriage, years filled with devotion and loyalty. These examples shaped my heart, instilling in me the deepest sense of what love can and should be. I knew one day I would find that kind of love, someone who would see me, cherish me, and build a life with me.

Years passed, filled with hopes, dreams, and waiting. I searched with an open heart, hoping to meet someone who saw love as I did, who longed for a family and a life woven together with care and devotion. I poured myself into my world, surrounding myself with family, friends, a fulfilling career, and adventures that took me to eleven countries. After much hesitation, I turned to online dating, Tinder, of all places. I had my doubts, wondering if anything true could come from it, but I told myself that if I stayed honest and true to my values, perhaps fate might surprise me. Then, in the most unexpected way, my world shifted.

Through a little twist of fate in the middle of a pandemic, I matched with Trevor. In a time when the world was turned upside down, two separate worlds collided. Before 2019, both of us had been living and working in California. He was a College Strength and Conditioning Coach in Los Angeles, and I was a Creative Director of a gaming company near Sacramento. When the pandemic disrupted our paths, my company moved to remote work, bringing me back to my hometown. Trevor's career also took a sudden turn as sports shut down, leading him to a new path as a skilled tradesman, ultimately landing us both in Reno, Nevada. On January 3, 2021, he made the move, and just a few weeks later, on January 30, we went on our first date. As we talked, I realized we shared a deep commitment to family, a belief in hard work, and a quiet determination. That evening marked the beginning of something extraordinary. From that moment on, we became inseparable, weaving our lives together with laughter, shared dreams, and the steady presence of true love.

As we settled into life together, we quickly filled our days with adventures and unforgettable memories. Whether it was camping in Mammoth Lakes, attending weddings and concerts, or just spending time with family and friends, each experience strengthened our connection. Things moved quickly in our relationship, and after only three months, we knew it was time to take the next step and move in together. Our love grew through the quiet and exciting moments, vacations, holidays, and simple days that felt bigger because we shared them. It was during these moments that I knew, more than ever, that we were building something real and lasting.

On a beautifully sunny day in San Diego, Trevor and I were at Mission Beach with my family. As we walked along the shoreline, searching for shells with the waves gently lapping at our feet, he took my hand and spun me toward him. Looking deeply into my eyes, he spoke about how much he loved me and how much he valued our communication, commitment, and the bond we'd built together. Then, he slowly dropped down on one knee.

Trevor opened a small navy blue velvet box, revealing the most beautiful, custom-designed emerald-cut diamond ring. He spoke the four words I had dreamt of my entire life, "Will you marry me?" Emotion flooded through me, I was overwhelmed with excitement, barely able to process that this was real. Stuck in a loop of happiness and surprise, I could only manage, "I can't even... I can't even..." as I nodded vigorously, my heart screaming yes. With a smile and tears in my eyes, he slid the ring onto my left hand, and on September 10, 2022, we were officially engaged.

Just six months later, on March 11, 2023, we were married at The Virgil in Reno, surrounded by family and friends who had supported and celebrated our love. The day was perfect, a traditional ceremony filled with joy, love, and the promise of forever. As I stood across from Trevor, holding his hands, I felt an overwhelming wave of gratitude and excitement.

When it came time to say our vows, we kept it simple and traditional, answering with the timeless "I do." Yet in my excitement, when it was my turn, I blurted out "Yes!" instead. It was such a sweet and funny moment, one that still makes me giggle every time I think back on it. It reminds me that life can still surprise us with unexpected laughter, even in the most prepared moments.

Our wedding day was everything I had dreamed of and more. It marked the beginning of our forever, a promise to face life's joys and challenges together. As we danced the night away surrounded by the people we love most, I felt a deep certainty that we could face anything life had in store with Trevor by my side.

Trevor is more than I ever imagined my prince charming could be. Each morning, I wake up next to him, filled with wonder that I get to love him for a lifetime. Every day, he makes me more grateful, more in love, and more certain that I have found my forever. He is a man of principles, determination, strength, protection, and intelligence. He has shown me a love so complete, so unshakeable, that I can barely find the words to describe it. He is more than the man I dreamed of as a little girl, the one who would see my heart, cherish me, and build a life with me. He is the man I want to raise our children, my partner, my best friend, and my reason for everything.

Every dream I have for the future is rooted alongside him. We look forward to a life filled with love, laughter, joy, and family. I vow to share my love with him for the rest of my days and beyond, forever grateful to be his and to call him mine.

CONCEPTION

Becoming a mother has been the most profound dream of my life, rooted in the deepest part of who I am. It's a dream I've carried for as long as I can remember, something I've always longed for. With Trevor by my side, that dream, the blessing of creating a family of our own, can finally become a beautiful reality.

After nearly a year of trying to conceive without success, we decided to seek help. Despite our best efforts, conceiving proved challenging, and we realized that our dream needed a little extra help. With hope in our hearts and a bit of nervous excitement, we decided to take the next step and were referred to the Nevada Center for Reproductive Medicine (NCRM).

We felt a sense of reassurance from the moment we walked into NCRM. The warmth and professionalism of the staff instantly put us at ease as we began a series of consultations and tests. The journey through fertility treatments is often described as an emotional rollercoaster, and for good reason, each step brings with it a mix of hope, anxiety, and perseverance.

Thankfully, all of our evaluations came back positive, with no significant concerns beyond a slight hormonal imbalance that was corrected after thirty days of medication. Having fertility assistance is a meticulously tracked and monitored process. Every step is timed, every hormone measured, every milestone planned. On February 29th, I received what is called a "trigger shot," a Human Chorionic Gonadotropin (hCG) injection. This crucial step stimulated the final maturation and release of the egg from my ovary. It felt like the beginning of something monumental, though we knew there was still much ahead.

The days following were filled with hope and cautious patience. Two weeks after the trigger shot, on March 19th, I went in for blood work to measure my hCG levels, the test that would tell us whether we were pregnant. After leaving the clinic, I kept my phone close, anxiously awaiting the results.

Later that day, the call came. I saw the voicemail notification pop up on my phone, and my heart skipped a beat. Trevor was at work, and we had promised to hear the news together. It took all my willpower not to listen to it right away. For hours, I carried my phone like a fragile treasure, resisting the urge to press play while anticipation bubbled up inside me.

When Trevor came home, he rushed through the door, his face filled with the same nervous excitement I felt. We didn't waste a second. Sitting side by side on the couch, I opened the voicemail and hit play.

"Hi, this is the Nevada Center for Reproductive Medicine. I have wonderful news: Congratulations! You're pregnant!"

The words filled the room, and for a moment, time seemed to stop. Tears welled up in my eyes as I turned to Trevor, who was already smiling so vastly that his happiness lit up the entire space. We didn't say much, we just held each other as the reality of the moment sank in.

The journey to parenthood is often depicted in movies as a moment of suspenseful anticipation, peeing on a stick, waiting for the test to reveal that elusive + sign, and then bursting into celebration. For us, the reality was far different but no less magical. It wasn't the cinematic scene of holding a pregnancy test in hand, but it was perfect in its own way. As we held each other and let the news sink in, I felt an immense wave of love, not just for the baby growing inside me but for the journey that had brought us here.

The rest of the day was a blur of emotions. We laughed, cried, and let our imaginations run wild with visions of the beautiful life we were about to create. The moment was a perfect blend of science, faith, and love, our unique story and one we would treasure forever.

Now, as we eagerly await the arrival of our precious baby, our hearts overflow with appreciation. The Nevada Center for Reproductive Medicine not only helped us achieve our dream but also gave us the greatest gift of all, the promise of a little life to cherish. Their dedication, compassion, and expertise have profoundly impacted our journey, and we will be forever thankful for their role in making our dream a reality.

We are due to welcome our beautiful baby into the world on November 23, 2024.

PREGNANCY

Pregnancy is an experience I hold close to my heart, there's something deeply primal, profound, and almost sacred about it. The miracle of creating life and nurturing a new soul feels like fulfilling my truest purpose, a beautiful gift to the world.

Every day, I felt a growing connection to the tiny life inside me. The first flutter of movement was like a whisper from our baby, a reassurance that they were there, growing and thriving. Seeing our baby on the ultrasound screen brought tears to my eyes every time, the way their tiny body wiggled, and their heart flickered with life was nothing short of miraculous. Each moment, each milestone, deepened the immense love and anticipation I felt for meeting our precious gift. It was as if I carried not just a child but a dream that was coming to life within me.

When we first found out we were expecting, we began discussing the importance of different delivery options and prenatal care. We weighed the pros and cons of each, considering the structured environment of a hospital, the personalized care of birthing centers, and the natural, hands-on approach of working with midwives. These conversations helped us align our priorities and values, ensuring we felt confident and supported throughout the birthing experience.

After extensive research, we decided to seek out a professional who could provide both medical care and emotional support. We were fortunate to find an incredible certified and licensed midwife who became an essential part of our journey. Her holistic approach prioritized my health, well-being, and maternal instincts, creating a space where we felt safe and celebrated every step of the way.

Alongside our midwife, I continued my routine prenatal visits at OB/GYN Associates. Having both a midwife and an obstetrician provided the ideal combination of nurturing care and comprehensive medical expertise. This dual approach gave us a strong foundation, helping us feel supported and informed. However, we soon learned that not every healthcare provider was open to this type of collaborative care.

During one of my routine prenatal visits at OB/GYN Associates, I eagerly shared my excitement about combining midwifery care with traditional obstetric care. My family has trusted this practice for three generations, which deepened my confidence in their care. However, the obstetrician's demeanor quickly changed, becoming visibly agitated as they declared that dual care was not permitted in their office. They even threatened to terminate me as a patient if I pursued this path. In an attempt to de-escalate the situation, I assured them that I was still weighing my options, hoping to proceed with the appointment. Reluctantly, they agreed to check my baby's heartbeat, but their comments left me shaken.

Throughout the rest of the appointment, their tone became increasingly critical. Warning me that midwifery care would significantly "increase the risk of fetal demise," going so far as to say it wasn't their responsibility to "clean up the mess created by a midwife." Their words were harsh and unyielding. They made it clear that if I pursued dual care, I would no longer be accepted as a patient at OB/GYN Associates, stating that no one in their practice would be willing to work with me if I continued down this path.

Their words stung deeply, but they also reinforced the importance of having a healthcare team that genuinely listens, respects, and values you as an individual. Despite this disheartening encounter, I remained steadfast in my determination to advocate for myself and my baby.

In contrast, midwifery care brought so much enjoyment and peace to our pregnancy journey. She monitored my baby's growth, taught us about the birthing process, and celebrated every milestone alongside us. This support, combined with Trevor's unwavering encouragement, gave me the strength to focus on the wonders of pregnancy.

Despite these challenges, I chose to focus on the positive aspects of my pregnancy. The journey was a balance of determination, self-advocacy, and love, woven together with highs and lows that made each milestone all the more meaningful.

One of the most exciting milestones was our Noninvasive Prenatal Testing (NIPT). This blood test analyzes small fragments of fetal DNA circulating in a pregnant woman's bloodstream. If Y-chromosome DNA is detected, the fetus is male; if no Y-chromosome DNA is detected, the fetus is female.

We anxiously waited nearly two weeks for the results to be posted online. I found myself hitting refresh almost hourly, unable to contain my anticipation. Finally, the results were posted. My heart racing, I blindly printed the page and placed it face down on the coffee table. Trevor and I sat side by side on the couch, holding hands as we prepared to discover the answer together.

With a mix of excitement and nervous energy, we eagerly flipped the paper over, our eyes frantically scanning the page. Then, we saw it, the word "Female." A flood of emotions washed over us as we hugged tightly, laughing and crying in equal measure. Knowing we were bringing a daughter into the world marked the beginning of a beautiful new chapter in our lives.

The closer we got to my due date, the more everything began to feel real. One moment stands out vividly in my mind, watching Trevor lovingly build our baby girl's crib. As I sat nearby, his focus and care brought tears to my eyes. Each piece he placed was a testament to his devotion to our growing family. Watching the nursery take shape felt like watching our dreams unfold, one thoughtful touch at a time. It wasn't just furniture coming together, it was the realization of how much love and intention had gone into this journey.

It feels like just yesterday that we were on our first date, learning about each other and dreaming about the future. From that moment to our wedding day, and now as we expect our first child together, every step of our journey has been a whirlwind of love and growth. Sitting there, watching Trevor with the same thoughtfulness and care he has always shown, I was reminded of how far we have come.

As the nursery came together, so did my emotions. Each day brought us closer to holding our daughter, and the anticipation filled me with overwhelming joy. Pregnancy wasn't just about carrying life, it was about preparing our hearts, our home, and our future for the incredible adventure ahead. Knowing that soon we would welcome our little one into this space, surrounded by so much love, made every moment even more special.

Each week brought us closer to meeting our baby girl, and with my husband's help, we planned our baby shower for July 20th, during my second trimester. Though some criticized our timing, calling it early by conventional standards, I brushed it off. I was eager to celebrate and ensure everything was ready for our little girl's arrival.

Hosting the shower early felt like the perfect choice for many reasons. For those who know me well, it is no surprise that I love to be organized and well-prepared. I've always valued staying ahead of the curve, so I wanted every detail to be in place long before her debut. Stories of early arrivals and unfinished nurseries only strengthened my resolve to stay ahead of schedule. Another important consideration was family, planning the shower during the summer months made it easier for loved ones to travel and allowed us to avoid Reno's unpredictable fall weather. Summer was the perfect season to celebrate new beginnings, surrounded by the people who mean the most to us. It gave us the freedom to focus on nesting and savoring the excitement of preparing for our sweet girl in the months ahead.

The day of the shower, held at Bundox Bocce, is everything we could hope for and more. Surrounded by family and friends, we laugh, share stories, and bask in the bliss of the moment. The room radiates love, filled with the presence of people who have supported us through so many seasons of life. Some traveled far and wide to be here, making the day even more special. Every smile, every hug, and every kind word feels like a gift, a beautiful reminder of how deeply our baby girl is already cherished.

As I look around the room, I am struck by the overwhelming sense of love I feel for this amazing community. These are the people who have celebrated our milestones, comforted us in tough times, and now stand beside us as we prepare for our greatest adventure yet, becoming parents. Their excitement for our little girl is incredibly grounding, offering reassurance that she will be welcomed into a circle of love and support.

As we left that day, my heart felt fuller than ever. The thought of our daughter growing up surrounded by such a remarkable community filled me with gratitude beyond words. It was more than just a celebration, it was a heartfelt reminder of the love that awaited her.

EMERGENCY

My life took an unexpected and frightening turn during a work trip from Reno, Nevada, to Cleveland, Ohio, for an eGaming Summit at Arrow International. On the morning of July 25th, around 6:00 am EST, I experienced emergency pregnancy complications at just 22 weeks gestation. As I was getting ready for work in the hotel room, I went to use the restroom when suddenly I felt a massive rush of water flood into the toilet, followed by significant bleeding. In an instant, I was thrown into the most terrifying and heartbreaking panic of my life.

As I frantically dove my hands into the overwhelming mix of blood and water, I was consumed by a desperate need to find my little girl. My mind raced with fear and disbelief, each second stretching into an eternity. The once-ordinary hotel room, where I had just been preparing for another day of work, now felt like a harrowing scene from which there was no escape. My heart pounded in my chest as I prayed for a miracle, hoping that I could somehow protect her from this overwhelming, cruel reality. The sheer helplessness I felt in that moment is something I will carry with me forever.

In shock and confusion, I quickly FaceTime Trevor, fumbling to get the words out. I kept asking, "What is happening? What is happening?" as I struggled to comprehend the gravity of the situation. My mind was racing, and I was overwhelmed by panic, unable to fully process what was going on.

In my frantic state, I hung up with Trevor and called our midwife, hoping for guidance and reassurance. As I described the symptoms, she calmly explained that I was most likely experiencing a miscarriage and needed to go to the hospital immediately, requiring urgent ambulance transport to MetroHealth Medical Center. Her words sent a chilling wave through me, underscoring the seriousness of the situation.

As I was boarded into the ambulance, I was hysterically crying, screaming, and pleading with every medical professional to check on my baby girl. However, they didn't have the necessary equipment until I was fully admitted to the Emergency Room. Once I arrived in the ER, they quickly hooked me up to a fetal monitor, poking and prodding me with various instruments. My heart skipped when I heard our baby girl's strong and steady heartbeat. It was the first moment of relief amidst the chaos.

After a vaginal exam and ultrasound, the obstetrician measured me to be 3.9 cm dilated and confirmed that my amniotic sac had ruptured, which was later discovered to be due to an infection called Chorioamnionitis after a placental pathology. This infection was affecting both me and the baby. The medical team acted swiftly, starting me on latency antibiotics to treat the Preterm Prelabor Rupture of Membranes (PPROM) to prevent maternal and fetal infections.

Thinking I was in active labor, they transferred me from the ER to the Labor & Delivery Unit, where I was hooked up to constant monitoring and multiple intravenous (IV) medications. The medical team administered fluids, magnesium, and two shots of antenatal betamethasone, a corticosteroid injection given to help my baby's lungs mature before birth. Despite the rupture, both my baby and placenta were still attached, and she continued to produce amniotic fluid on her own, which was a good sign. It indicated that she was growing and that her kidneys were functioning properly. Amazingly, she seemed unaffected, happily growing bigger and stronger as if nothing had happened.

After 12 long hours in the Labor & Delivery Unit, the doctors confirmed that I was not in active labor. They moved me to the Antepartum Unit, a lower-risk room, where I was placed on strict bed rest. It was one of the longest days I have ever experienced. Alone and scared, I missed my family more than I could ever put into words. Trevor, along with my mom and dad, endured 13 agonizing hours of travel, navigating multiple layovers and connections, to be by my side. When they finally walked into my room, it was as if the weight of the world had been lifted off my shoulders. Their embrace brought me the comfort and strength I so desperately needed, reminding me that even in the darkest moments, I was not alone.

During my hospitalization, I was faced with the heavy reality of our situation. Our daughter was only 22 weeks along, and the doctors came to us with somber expressions, carefully explaining the challenges we were up against. They spoke of potential complications, outlining the risks and possible outcomes with a delicacy that made the situation feel even more intense. Words like "severe preterm birth," "infections," "limited lung development," "brain bleeds," and "survival odds" came into the conversation, each one feeling like a weight pressing on my heart.

They prepared us for all the frightening possibilities, painting a picture of just how fragile her journey might be.

Every statistic and every caution they provided was meant to protect us, yet each one felt like a blow to my hopes. I could sense the challenge of what was to come, and all I could do was hold on tightly to whatever strength I had left. Despite the odds stacked against her, I remained determined to stay hopeful. Despite all the uncertainty, I knew our sweet baby girl was already a fighter, and together, we would face every single day, hour, and minute with unwavering love and support.

Every heartbeat, every wiggle, every scan became a lifeline, a reminder that despite the odds stacked against us, she was holding on. Each morning began with a fetal monitoring session, and I clung to the sound of her heartbeat as though it were the melody keeping me grounded. On good days, it beat strong and steady, a reassurance that she was thriving in the face of impossible odds. On other days, when her heartbeat dipped, or monitoring stretched longer than planned, the fear crept in, testing my strength and faith.

Over the course of seven days, both my sweet baby girl and I have been stable. The medical team monitors her heart once a day for 20 minutes, and the plan is to continue the pregnancy while I remain hospitalized on strict bed rest, ensuring she grows as much as possible. With each passing day, her odds of survival grow stronger. The goal is to reach 34 weeks gestation, though her arrival ultimately depends on her. If contractions begin, we hope for a natural delivery, but any signs of distress or changes in either of our heart rates will necessitate an emergency C-section. Once she is born, she will go straight to the Neonatal Intensive Care (NICU) for immediate care and remain there until she reaches full term or is strong enough to be discharged.

We've heard many inspiring stories and focus on the positives as much as possible. MetroHealth is recognized as one of the top hospitals in the country, in the top 98th percentile nationwide. We believe it's God's plan for us to be here, and we trust that everything is as it should be. We're taking it day by day, and every day is a victory.

BIRTH

By the morning of August 1st, after eight long days confined to strict bed rest, the weight of immobility began to settle heavily on my body, making me acutely aware of its toll. The lack of movement brought on various aches and pains, most notably an unrelenting discomfort in my lower back and digestive system. I reported the pain to my doctors, who immediately grew concerned. They explained that lower back pain could be an early sign of labor. They quickly connected me to a fetal monitor, and I spent an anxious hour listening to the steady rhythm of my baby's heartbeat. When the results returned normal with no signs of contractions, labor was ruled out, providing a brief moment of relief.

As the day continued, I started experiencing intense cramping, coupled with a sense of urgency to use the restroom. Convinced it was nothing more than constipation, the doctors administered medication to alleviate the issue. For a short time, it seemed to work, the cramping eased, and I dared to hope that the worst had passed. I stood up to head to the restroom, but just as I took a step, an overwhelming sensation of pressure between my legs stopped me in my tracks. Instinctively, I crossed my legs and urgently called out to Trevor, "Call the doctor! Call the doctor!"

Within moments, the high-risk obstetrician rushed in, performing a thorough examination. To my relief, she confirmed no changes in dilation or the baby's position. Her reassurances helped calm my nerves, even as I continued to feel the persistent cramping and pressure. I was determined to believe that everything was fine.

Nearly an hour passed before I summoned the courage to approach the bathroom again, only to feel that overwhelming pressure return, stronger and more urgent than before. Suddenly, instinct took over, and I cradled my hands beneath me just in time to feel her tiny head crowning. Time seemed to freeze. In the midst of chaos, Trevor and I stood there in stunned silence as we realized our baby girl was being born. It was as if the world faded away, and there was a serene stillness in its place. Despite the terrifying circumstances, an inexplicable wave of calm washed over us.

With one gentle, instinctual push, she was here, our baby girl, cradled in my hands. Trevor and I stared in awe at the tiny miracle before us. For a fleeting moment, it was just the three of us, suspended in the quiet beauty of her arrival. Then reality surged back as we shouted, 'She's here! She's here!' Within seconds, the nurse rushed into the room, her urgency matching the gravity of the moment. Yet, for that brief, unforgettable instant, time stood still, and we were alone, marveling at the life we had brought into the world.

She cried as she took her first breath, breathing on her own and eliminating any urgent medical attention or resuscitation, defying the grim predictions that had loomed over us. That first sound filled the room with a glimmer of hope, sending relief and joy coursing through Trevor and me, as well as the medical staff who had been bracing for the worst. It was a collective exhale, a moment that reaffirmed the belief that maybe, just maybe, she could beat the odds.

In a whirlwind, the world came back into focus. Nearly 20 staff members, including nurses and doctors, flooded into the room. They clamped our baby girl's umbilical cord, and Trevor—now officially "Dad"—cut the cord. Then, in a flash, the care team whisked our baby girl to the neonatal bassinet in the room, an OmniBed known as a Giraffe Warmer, where they worked to ensure her tiny body was stable.

Meanwhile, I was gently guided back to bed to deliver the placenta. Trevor seemed to be everywhere at once, by her side, watching over her with a fierce protectiveness and back by mine, holding my hand and whispering words of comfort as the doctors tended to me. His strength anchored me in those overwhelming moments, a steady presence in a sea of activity.

Once the placenta was delivered, I was placed on a two-hour hold to monitor for hemorrhaging, preventing me from immediately following our baby girl to the NICU. It was agonizing to stay behind, but I found solace knowing Trevor was with her every step of the way. As I lay there, the realization of what had just transpired began to sink in. Our baby girl had entered the world with grace and determination all on her own, and the love surrounding her was already immeasurable.

When I finally joined them in the NICU, seeing Trevor by her side, protective and tender, filled my heart with profound gratitude. Our journey had taken an unexpected turn, but at that moment, I knew that together, we were ready to face whatever came next. We were a family.

NICU

Zoya Pari Robinson

August 1, 2024

6:43 PM PST

1 lb 8 oz | 11.42"

23 weeks, 5 days

We are overjoyed to welcome our beautiful daughter into the world! On August 1, 2024, at just 23 weeks and 5 days gestation, Zoya Pari Robinson entered the world. She was impossibly small, weighing only 1 pound 8 ounces, yet in that tiny body lived a spirit far greater than her size.

Zoya's first breaths came with a sweet determination that took everyone by surprise. We had been warned about the risks, the challenges, and the terrifying unknowns of the potential complications that come with a micro preemie. The doctors had prepared us for the worst, failure to breathe, the imminent need for resuscitation, and the heartbreak of watching her slip away. Yet, instead, she fought back with every breath, pushing through with the kind of strength that no one expected from a baby so small, tiny, vulnerable, and fragile. That first cry told us something, this is no ordinary baby, she is a fighter.

From the moment Zoya entered this world, she demonstrated what an incredible miracle she is, amazing everyone around her. Her first assessment of life called an APGAR score, shocked medical professionals. The APGAR test is a quick evaluation of a newborn's health conducted at one, five, and ten minutes after birth. It measures five key criteria: Appearance (skin color), Pulse (heart rate), Grimace response (reflexes), Activity (muscle tone), and Respiration (breathing effort), with a maximum total score of 10. Despite her extreme prematurity, Zoya scored an astonishing 7 at one minute, improving to 9 at five and ten minutes. These scores are exceptionally high for a baby born so early, a testament to her incredible strength and will to survive.

In shock, we are caught between the raw joy of her arrival and the crushing fear of what lies ahead. It is unimaginable. Every time a nurse or doctor enters the room, it was as if a new wave of anxiety washed over us. Zoya's tiny body is hooked up to more machines than I can count, her frame hardly big enough to fit all the medical sensors, and each one seems to scream at us, reminding us just how delicate she is.

Her skin, as thin as paper, bore the weight of every attachment, each one a sacrifice to its integrity.

The NICU is both suffocating and full of tenuous hope. Every second feels like an eternity. It is a world where time seems to bend. Trevor and I stand by her side, but the isolation is overwhelming. We are here, but Zoya is fighting alone in ways we can't fully comprehend. I can't comfort her directly, can't ease her pain, but I'm here, wishing I could do more, hold her, kiss her, and cradle her in my arms. We are learning to find strength in the quiet moments, her tiny fingers gripping mine, the steady rhythm of her breath, and the sound of the machines that keep her going. In this bleak, isolating place, these fleeting glimpses of connection are the threads that hold us together.

This new reality is a world of its own, a place of constant ambiguity. The sterile walls of the unit have become our home, and the hum of machines is now the rhythm of our daily lives. CP4-141 is our new address, confined to this small, 12-by-12 room, its glass walls a constant reminder of how our lives have been swallowed whole by the NICU. Yet, this isn't just a place for medical care, it is where our family's story begins, where we discover strength in the most unlikely of places.

We are thousands of miles from home, a place that feels more like a dream we can't wake up from. The life we once knew, our family, our friends, our home, and our jobs, feels like a distant memory, something we can't quite reach, like a fading photograph tucked in a forgotten drawer. It all seems so far away, yet we carry it with us in quiet moments when the bustle of the hospital fades, and all we have left is each other.

Everything we've ever known has been left behind, and in its place, we've found a new world, a world where the tiny, fragile life of our daughter consumes our every waking thought and breath. It's hard to explain the magnitude of this shift, how everything that once felt important has shifted in weight, and how our entire existence has become about this small being fighting so hard to thrive. The world no longer binds us outside these glass walls. We've let it all go, knowing that if we had to, we would let the whole world crumble around us. Nothing else matters now, nothing but being here, with Zoya, holding on to hope, love, and faith, knowing she needs us here more than anything.

Zoya is named in honor of my great-grandmother Zoja Pari (pronounced Zo·ya), a woman whose unwavering strength and resilience shaped the very foundation of our family. We believe that Zoja's spirit lives on in our little girl, watching over her as a guardian angel. The name Zoya has Greek origins, meaning "life," though its spelling and pronunciation may vary across cultures, its universal symbolism of vitality and endurance remains constant. During WWII, Zoja's bravery was tested as she escaped Estonia with her two young daughters, navigating war-torn Europe to ensure their survival. Just as Zoja protected her daughters during this perilous time, we believe her enduring spirit will guide and protect our little Zoya throughout her life. In this way, Zoya doesn't just carry the name of her great-great-grandmother, she carries her legacy, a legacy of survival, strength, and a fierce love for life.

This is not a journey we expected, but Zoya's fight teaches us what true resilience means. We wouldn't want to be anywhere else but by her side, believing in her strength and knowing she will overcome this. She is our miracle, and we will keep fighting for her every second of every day. She is showing us how to be strong, how to survive, and how to love fiercely. We will never stop fighting, not for a second.

Our precious daughter, her dad, and I will remain in the Level III Neonatal Intensive Care Unit at MetroHealth Medical Center in Cleveland, Ohio, under the care of a dedicated medical team. She will stay here until she is full-term or has gained enough strength to be discharged.

AUGUST

In Zoya's first moments of life, she was carefully placed into a temperature-controlled isolette, a specialized incubator designed to provide a stable and protective environment for her tiny, delicate body. This remarkable device ensured that her body temperature remained consistent, mimicking the warmth of the womb while shielding her from outside stresses. Alongside the isolette, a pulse oximeter was placed to continuously monitor her oxygen levels and heart rate, and three electrocardiogram (ECG) leads were attached to track her vital signs in real time, providing the medical team with crucial insights into her condition.

In those critical early hours, thin medical tubes called umbilical arterial catheters (UAC) became Zoya's lifelines. Inserted into the vessels of her umbilical cord, these catheters provided a direct path for delivering vital fluids, medications, and nutrients into her tiny body. They also allowed doctors to monitor her blood gases and draw samples without causing her unnecessary distress, a crucial step in preserving her fragile strength. Alongside the isolette, pulse oximeter, and monitoring leads, the UAC formed part of a delicate, life-sustaining system, working tirelessly to support Zoya's underdeveloped organs and give her the best possible chance to grow and thrive in her earliest days.

Zoya was immediately placed on Total Parenteral Nutrition (TPN), a vital necessity for premature babies unable to tolerate full enteral feeding. TPN provides her with the essential macro and micronutrients she needs to grow and develop, carefully tailored to meet her specific needs. The NICU team manages her nutrition with incredible precision, adjusting her electrolytes, vitamins, and minerals daily to support her fragile system. They monitor her blood work multiple times a day to ensure her levels remain within a safe range, keeping a close eye on any deficiencies or imbalances. Additionally, her blood gases are checked frequently to track her CO_2 levels and assess her lung function, ensuring she receives the right amount of respiratory support. The level of diligence and care given to her tiny body was nothing short of extraordinary, a testament to the dedication of her medical team in helping her thrive.

Zoya began facing her initial challenges as the first few days unfolded. Before her birth, the doctors painted a sobering picture of the obstacles she might encounter with an underdeveloped system, fragile lungs, and the looming threat of relentless infections. Each word carried the weight of uncertainty, a storm of possibilities that could shatter her fragile grip on life. Every second felt like standing on the edge of a cliff, holding our breath, praying the ground beneath her would hold firm against the chaos threatening to pull her away. Among those concerns were the risks to her heart and brain, which are serious issues in severely premature babies.

The doctors explained the critical need to evaluate her heart's function and rule out any complications. In her first days of life, a heart echocardiogram was ordered to assess her cardiac performance, filling pressure, and hemodynamics. They also screened for patent ductus arteriosus (PDA), a condition where a blood vessel near the heart fails to close properly after birth, leading to significant complications. At the same time, they performed a cranial ultrasound (CrUS) to check for bleeding or abnormalities in her brain, knowing that preemies are especially vulnerable to such conditions.

Filled with uncertainty and fear, we anxiously awaited the results. Thankfully, Zoya's tests brought us the best news we could hope for, her heart was strong, and her brain ultrasound revealed no significant issues. The only finding was a slight grade 1 germinal matrix hemorrhage similar to a bruise, which the doctors assured us would heal naturally over the next couple of months. That moment of relief was profound, a small yet significant triumph in what often felt like an endless fight for her health and future.

As we continued to navigate these early days, Zoya began facing new challenges. After 72 hours of life, her tiny yet mighty body worked tirelessly to breathe, but her underdeveloped lungs struggle to expel enough CO_2, requiring additional support. To help her, the doctors transition her from her conventional ventilator to an oscillator, a specialized ventilator designed to deliver very small, rapid breaths. This machine helps preemies like Zoya maintain steady lung expansion while minimizing the risk of lung injury, giving her fragile lungs the support they need to rest and heal.

Yet, as quickly as these interventions begin, Zoya shows us her incredible strength. After just 48 hours on the oscillator, she responds positively and is transitioned back to the conventional ventilator. As these initial days draw to a close, we celebrate a milestone that fills our hearts with hope. After just 13 days, Zoya is extubated, a remarkable achievement by any medical standard considering her gestational age.

Breathing more independently, she amazes us with her unwavering determination to grow stronger each day.

After nearly two weeks, Zoya's umbilical catheters are carefully removed, marking an essential step in her progress. These have been crucial for blood sampling, blood pressure monitoring, and delivering the TPN that sustains her in her earliest days. To maintain her care, the doctors place a peripherally inserted central catheter (PICC) through a vein in her leg, carefully threading it up to her heart. This new line now serves as her lifeline, enabling the precise delivery of medications and nutrients while minimizing infection risks and supporting her ongoing recovery.

We've had to adapt quickly to this unfamiliar world, finding joy in milestones many parents might overlook. Every day has brought a rhythm of small yet extraordinary progress: her first 'poop,' her first tentative smile, and swabbing her tiny mouth with breast milk, a way of nurturing her when holding or feeding her wasn't yet possible. When her umbilical cord fell off, it revealed the tiniest, sweetest belly button we had ever seen, a detail so small, yet it symbolized her growth and the progress she was making. That same week, she opened her eyes for the first time, her bright, curious gaze taking in the world around her. It was as if she were meeting us in a new way, and with every blink, our connection deepened.

Every interaction, no matter how small, felt monumental. With care limited to just four times a day, every six hours, those moments of connection became our only way to touch and care for our beautiful baby.

A moment we had dreamed of for so long finally arrived, we held Zoya for the very first time. As her tiny body rested against mine, her warmth seeped into my soul, melting away what seemed like an eternity of fear and uncertainty. The world outside the NICU faded, leaving only the profound connection between us and our daughter. I wept as I held her, not from sadness but from the overwhelming gratitude and love that filled me. That moment was a promise, a promise that no matter how long this journey took, we would walk it together.

Now, as Zoya approaches one month old, her doctor notices a change in her demeanor, signaling the onset of an illness. Battling this infection and severe anemia, she requires immediate antibiotics and her first blood transfusion. The combination of fluctuating CO_2 levels and anemia leaves her visibly exhausted, hcr nearly translucent skin a stark reflection of how critically low her blood supply has become. With a total volume of just 40-50 mL, equivalent to only three to four tablespoons, every milliliter lost feels like a precious sacrifice.

In the face of her severe anemia, we learn that Zoya has type A positive blood, the same type as mine. As soon as I know she needs blood, I don't hesitate to offer my own. However, despite the sincerity of my offer, it cannot be accepted. The stringent cleaning process required for donor blood given to premature babies renders mine unsuitable. Fortunately, the hospital's donor program provides a lifesaving match with a single blood donor who will remain matched with her for any future transfusions. This ensures that each transfusion is perfectly compatible, serving as a crucial source of stability for her fragile system. Nearly immediately, her transfusion improves her vitals, and her determined little spirit starts to shine through.

To further support her fragile blood supply, Zoya's doctors introduce Darbepoetin, a medication designed to stimulate the production of red blood cells and reduce the need for transfusions. This treatment gives her body the chance to take a more active role in her recovery. The best part? It was working.

It isn't long before Zoya triumphs over both the infection and anemia, adding them both to the growing list of challenges she has already conquered. Her happy, alert self returns, and her feisty nature is on full display as she waves her tiny arms with unmistakable determination.

From the moment Zoya was born, I was fortunate with the ability to produce breastmilk right away, a rare occurrence for mothers of preemies. The hormonal signals that stimulate milk production typically develop later in pregnancy, closer to full term, making this an incredibly special and unexpected gift. Driven by an overwhelming determination to give her the best possible start in life, I immediately began pumping to ensure she would have a steady supply of milk ready for the day she could finally feed.

After weeks of Zoya relying exclusively on TPN, her tiny body grows stable enough to transition to a nasogastric (NG) tube, a thin, flexible tube inserted through her nose and into her stomach. This milestone allows her to finally receive my breastmilk, a lifeline of nourishment uniquely designed to meet her fragile needs. Rich in vital nutrients, immune-boosting components, and growth-promoting properties, breastmilk not only sustains her but also supports the development of her intestinal tract and helps establish a healthy gut biome, essential for her overall growth and long-term health. The ability to provide such an extraordinary source of nutrition to my baby girl feels like a profound and deeply personal connection with her.

One of the brightest milestones on this journey comes when Zoya attempts non-nutritive latching for the first time. Though she is still too young to feed orally, this practice, where she instinctively latches and sucks without drawing milk, helps prepare her for breastfeeding in the future. Watching her tiny mouth open eagerly, practicing the delicate coordination of sucking, swallowing, and breathing, fills us with awe. At that moment, it feels as though all the effort and love poured into providing her with milk is coming full circle, a step toward the day she will feed on her own.

We marvel at how much she has achieved in just her first month of life. She is a warrior with the heart of a champion. Yet, just as things seem to calm, Zoya faces new challenges.

SEPTEMBER

We are navigating some of the most harrowing moments of our lives, testing us in ways we never imagined. Zoya is braving one of her toughest battles yet, a diagnosis of Necrotizing Enterocolitis (NEC) and a Cytomegalovirus (CMV) infection. Each condition carries profound risks, especially for a preemie as tiny and fragile as our baby girl.

NEC, a severe intestinal disease that primarily affects premature infants, causes inflammation in the bowel that can lead to tissue death. In the most severe cases, it results in perforations in the intestines, allowing bacteria to leak into the abdomen and bloodstream, causing life-threatening infections. Early signs on Zoya's X-rays reveal abnormal gas patterns consisting of a bubbly appearance in the walls of her intestines. The medical team responds swiftly, administering antibiotics to combat NEC and halting her feeds to give her intestines the rest they desperately need. This condition hangs heavily over us, its severity threatening not only her immediate health but also her long-term ability to absorb nutrients and grow. The fragility of her tiny body feels painfully tangible, making every moment a test of her strength and the team's expertise.

Despite the gravity of these diagnoses, Zoya's spirit remains unyielding. Within just 48 hours, her symptoms improved so rapidly that her doctors began questioning whether the NEC diagnosis was accurate. Her remarkable progress has left the medical team astonished and filled our hearts with renewed hope. Yet, even as uncertainty surrounds one battle, another remains clear, Zoya is fighting CMV, a condition that tests her resilience further.

Cytomegalovirus (CMV) infection is a common but potentially life-threatening virus for premature infants with underdeveloped immune systems. In Zoya's case, the CMV infection leads to complications in her gastrointestinal tract, a condition known as CMV Colitis, a serious complication that inflames her gastrointestinal tract and heightens her susceptibility to additional infections. Quantitative viral load testing confirms the diagnosis, giving her medical team the clarity they need to tailor her treatment plan. CMV severely weakens her defenses, leading to critically low platelet levels, a condition worsened by the antiviral medication Ganciclovir, which is essential for fighting the infection but comes with significant risks, including potential impacts on her hearing, vision, and neurological development. To stabilize her condition, Zoya undergoes six platelet transfusions and an additional blood transfusion throughout her infection, each one a vital effort to counteract the risk of spontaneous bleeding. Despite the complexities and challenges of her care, Zoya's resilience shines through, inspiring hope as she continues to fight this relentless virus.

With Zoya's diagnoses and the immediate halt of her feeds, my milk supply began to decline. The emotional toll of watching her battle these life-threatening conditions started to wear me thin. The stress, anxiety, and helplessness I felt made it increasingly difficult to maintain the rigorous pumping schedule I had so carefully followed. Zoya's nutrition once again depended entirely on TPN, her fragile system sustained by meticulously calibrated infusions. It was heartbreaking to know that my milk, something I had poured so much energy and love into, was no longer a part of her care. Adding to this heartbreak was the realization that I might never experience the connection of breastfeeding her, as my supply continued to diminish.

Yet, even through the pain and exhaustion, I managed to pump enough milk to sustain her for nearly six months. The stock I built up became a lifeline, ensuring she could continue to receive the benefits of my milk even as her care shifted. Though I could no longer provide milk for her daily, I reminded myself that my role as her mother went beyond this single act. Whether through my milk, my advocacy, or simply standing by her side, my priority remained to support her in any way I could. Knowing that she would continue to receive the nourishment I had worked so hard to provide for months to come brought me a sense of comfort and peace during this incredibly challenging time.

It is nearly indescribable to convey the whirlwind of emotions we experience with every passing moment, enduring procedures, and treatments beyond what we ever thought one so small could bear. Every day, we watch her endure the endless pokes, prods, and procedures. Needle after needle, blood draw after blood draw, her delicate skin bruising with each prick. I stand by her bedside, tears streaming down my face, wishing with all my heart that I could take her place, that I could spare her this pain. She is so innocent, so little, and has already faced challenges so big. It's a helpless feeling, standing by, watching her flinch and tremble with each new procedure, yet there's nothing I can do to take it all away. All I want is to hold her close, to shield her from the world, but instead, I am separated by a thin barrier of acrylic, her isolette the only thing keeping her tiny body warm and safe. I stand there, helpless, watching as the doctors and nurses work tirelessly to heal her, longing for the day when I can finally cradle her in my arms without fear.

No matter how many tubes are attached or how many blood draws she endures, she keeps fighting. She's taught me what real strength looks like. In the moments when I'm at my lowest, ready to crumble, I look at her, and I find hope. Zoya's resilience gives me the strength to keep going and the unwavering belief that we will get through this together. She is our warrior, filling us with hope and purpose each day.

OCTOBER

Zoya reaches an incredible milestone, she is moving from her isolette to a crib. For months, her isolette has been her cocoon, a carefully controlled environment designed to replicate the warmth and protection of the womb. It maintains her fragile body at a stable temperature, shielding her from the world and giving her the time to grow stronger. Now, as her tiny systems mature and her ability to regulate her own temperature improves, this move feels like a monumental victory, proof of her growing independence.

This transition also changes everything for us as her parents. No longer separated by the isolette's acrylic walls, we finally have full, unrestricted access to her. For the first time, we can pick her up without waiting for permission or assistance, hold her close whenever we want, and shower her with endless kisses. This newfound freedom allows for unlimited bonding, the kind we have dreamed of since her birth. Gone are the days of peering through a transparent barrier, feeling both connected and apart from her. Now, she's truly in our arms, entirely ours to cradle, comfort, and love without limits.

Seeing her nestled in a crib for the first time is overwhelming in the best possible way. It's a moment that symbolizes so much more than just a change in equipment, it's a visual representation of how far she has come. No longer encased in a protective bubble of acrylic, she now looks like a baby ready for the world, free to stretch out and sleep in a space that feels less clinical and more like home. It's the first time we genuinely imagine her lying in her crib at home, snuggled in the nursery we've dreamed of for her.

The emotional weight of this milestone is immense. The crib feels like a bridge, carrying us from the distressing days of the NICU toward the light of normalcy. Unassisted by a temperature-controlled isolette, each breath she takes is a testament to the strength she has built over the past weeks and months. This simple yet profound moment fills us with a renewed sense of hope. It feels like the NICU journey inches closer to its end, and for the first time, the dream of bringing her home doesn't feel so far away.

Yet, even as she grows stronger, she faces another hurdle, a severe bacterial infection called Cellulitis in her hand, caused by the infiltration of an IV. This condition spreads quickly through the skin and deeper tissues, posing a significant risk if not treated urgently. Her tiny hand becomes swollen and red, prompting immediate action from her medical team. The infection is severe enough to require surgery to drain the affected area and reduce the risk of complications. Watching her endure this procedure is nerve-wracking, knowing how delicate her tiny body is and how much she has endured. Yet, true to her nature, Zoya faces it with quiet strength. After the surgery, the medical team starts her on antibiotics to ensure the infection doesn't spread further. Her body responds well, and the swelling begins to subside within days. Each step of her recovery reinforces just how extraordinary her spirit truly is.

As part of her comprehensive care in the NICU, Zoya undergoes regular screenings for Retinopathy of Prematurity (ROP). This condition poses a risk of blindness in premature babies due to abnormal blood vessel growth in the retina. Every two weeks, a specialized ophthalmologist carefully examines her developing eyes. These frequent check-ups are crucial for early detection and intervention, ensuring that potential issues can be addressed promptly. Thanks to the extraordinary diligence of her medical team, Zoya's eyes continue to develop normally, with no signs of ROP, a reassuring victory in her journey of overcoming challenges.

Progress continues steadily. Her airflow support is reduced as she transitions from the conventional ventilator to Vapotherm. This shift is significant, moving from invasive to non-invasive support not only allows her tiny lungs to continue developing but also reduces the stress on her fragile body. The heated, humidified oxygen delivered through Vapotherm keeps her airways comfortable and open, making each breath less of a struggle. Watching her breathe more independently feels like our time in the NICU is slowly but surely coming to a close.

On Halloween, we playfully celebrate her strength and spirit, dressing her as the 'prisoner of the NICU,' complete with a tiny ball and chain. The staff laugh and smile, their enjoyment reflecting how deeply Zoya touches their hearts. Each moment is precious, a little piece of normalcy in a world turned upside down.

NOVEMBER

As Zoya nears her original due date, her progress is undeniable, but one persistent challenge has defined much of her NICU journey, her dangerously low phosphorus levels. Despite the neonatologists and nutritionists carefully managing her macro and micronutrients with extraordinary precision, her phosphorus remains stubbornly low. She is receiving twice the recommended dose of sodium phosphate to support her growth and development, yet her levels refuse to reach the normal range. This ongoing struggle baffles her medical team and underscores the complexity of her condition, adding another layer to her fight for stability.

Zoya's journey with her phosphorus levels has become an all-encompassing mystery, one that sends shockwaves through her care team and pulls in specialists from the Mayo Clinic, Cleveland Clinic, and multiple other hospitals. Week after week, her bloodwork shows dangerously low phosphorus levels, a vital mineral for her growth and development. Without enough phosphorus, the body is forced to compensate by stealing calcium from the bones, a survival mechanism that can lead to significant long-term impacts on bone density and growth. The concern among her care team grows with every passing day.

The doctors begin consulting specialists to rule out every possible cause. An Infectious Disease doctor investigates whether her low phosphorus might be related to her CMV infection, which has already weakened her immune system. Next, an Endocrinologist examines her hypothyroidism to confirm her thyroid is functioning properly. When those tests reveal no abnormalities, a Nephrologist joins the team to investigate her kidneys, which, thankfully, are healthy. Despite the collective expertise of these specialists, no one can pinpoint why Zoya's phosphorus remains so critically low.

Zoya doesn't fit neatly into any diagnostic box. Every specialist reviews her case, consults their resources, and ultimately comes to the same conclusion, she is simply too premature. Her tiny body, they explain, is still growing stronger, and her organs are continuing to develop. They reassure us that, in time, she will likely grow out of this. Yet their words do little to ease our fear about the long-term effects this could have on her growth and development, especially as we learn more about the risks of prolonged low phosphorus levels.

The medical team's determination to leave no stone unturned leads them to test her genetics. A Hypophosphatemia Rickets Panel is ordered, a rare and comprehensive test that searches for genetic mutations linked to low phosphorus levels. The wait for results stretches into a long, agonizing month. For thirty days, we hold our breath, fear the unknown, and wonder what this could mean for her future. When the results finally come back, they show no abnormalities. While the relief is overwhelming, the question of why still lingers.

During this critical time, Zoya's medical team continues to address her dangerously low phosphorus levels with an intravenous phosphorus and calcium infusion. This treatment carries significant risks, as failure to properly monitor the calcium IV can cause severe damage to her skin and tissues. The stakes are high, and we are terrified of the potential consequences. A communication order is issued by the attending doctor, demanding continuous supervision of the IV to ensure it is monitored closely. However, despite the critical nature of the situation, some dismiss this vital communication order, which only increases our concern for her safety and well-being.

The stress is compounded by the fact that Zoya has already endured so many IVs, along with five failed attempts to place a secondary PICC line. Each failed attempt leaves her fragile veins further compromised. As the weeks pass, she is down to her last usable vein, adding a sense of urgency and fear to an already intense situation. Every additional procedure feels like it is pushing her to the edge, and we know that if this last vein fails, there might be no other options left.

Watching her endure such painful procedures leaves us feeling powerless, our frustration compounded by the negligence of a couple of staff members who ignored the doctor's communication orders. The emotional toll of ensuring her safety while advocating for her needs adds to the unbearable weight of the situation. At that moment, we truly understand how fragile and precarious Zoya's fight for survival is, and we are reminded of the overwhelming responsibility that comes with being a parent in the NICU.

Then, almost miraculously, Zoya's phosphorus levels began to rise. One week, her numbers reached the normal range for the first time, and they stayed there. For over a month now, her phosphorus levels have remained stable, a milestone we once feared might never arrive. It is as though her tiny body has decided it is ready to take this step forward, a testament to her incredible endurance.

Her medical team now refers to her condition as infant hypophosphatemia, degenerative bone disease, a diagnosis that sounds daunting but is expected to self-resolve within a few months. What once felt like an insurmountable battle has turned into a testament to her strength and how far she has come in her development. Zoya's story is one of relentless determination, not just from her doctors, who explore every avenue to ensure her health, but from Zoya, who defies every challenge with quiet, unyielding courage.

She is our warrior, our miracle, and our greatest inspiration. Every step forward reminds us of the immense challenges she has faced and the incredible progress she has made. Her journey may not fit into a box, but it is uniquely hers and nothing short of extraordinary.

DECEMBER

Zoya's stability brings a much-needed sense of relief. It feels as though the hardest days are finally behind us, allowing us to focus on the light ahead, bringing our sweet girl home. Each day, her vitals remain steady, and her care team speaks more frequently about discharge plans. The hope we've held onto for so long now feels more tangible, more real. For the first time, we can imagine life outside the hospital walls.

As Zoya's discharge draws near, we can't help but reflect on the bonds we formed with her primary nurses, who have become an inseparable part of our story. Their unwavering care, kindness, and expertise carried us through some of our darkest days. They weren't just caregivers, they became a part of our family. While we are overjoyed to start this new chapter at home, we will miss their comforting presence and the support they provided not just to Zoya, but to us as parents. They will always hold a special place in our hearts as a vital part of Zoya's journey.

The hospital became our universe, a microcosm of constant vigilance and unwavering hope. In that world, there were no real distinctions between day and night. The fluorescent lights were perpetual, casting a pale glow that became the backdrop to our every moment. The rhythms of life were dictated not by sunrise or sunset but by the sound of alarms, the shuffle of nurses' feet, and the rotation of care teams. Each shift brought new faces, updates, challenges, and prayers. Days and nights melded into one unending continuum, where time was marked only by Zoya's progress and setbacks.

The outside world became a distant memory. We stopped noticing the changing weather, the passing holidays, or the rhythms of everyday life. Inside those walls, life was frozen yet achingly alive. Every decision, every step, every ounce of energy poured into one singular focus, Zoya. This all-encompassing routine became our reality, and though it often felt suffocating, it also gave us purpose. In those moments, we clung to every small victory, every sign of growth, as a reminder that this chapter, though grueling, would one day come to an end.

In Zoya, we see not just a survivor but a warrior, reminding us that even the smallest among us can overcome the greatest challenges with grace and grit. As Zoya fights her battles with fortitude and perseverance, the toll it takes on us as her parents is immeasurable. Living in the hospital for 149 days, nearly five months, becomes a world of endless stimulation, a relentless barrage of beeps, dings, and alarms that echo through every corner of our lives. The moments we crave peace are constantly interrupted by the hum of activity: nurses changing shifts, doctors making rounds, specialists bringing updates, and a steady stream of voices and footsteps that never truly fade.

Every second feels filled with some kind of disruption, leaving no space for stillness or solace. Even the joy of Zoya's milestones, those moments we long to celebrate as a family, is robbed of its intimacy. There is no space to hold these precious memories close, they are shared with over a hundred nurses, doctors, and staff who always seem to know everything about her before we do. It feels as though our most precious moments with her are always shared, leaving us longing for a sense of privacy we can't seem to find.

Our lives become an open book, constantly on display for strangers who have access to every detail, every decision, and every piece of our daughter's fragile journey. It isn't just the physical confinement to a hospital room, it is the loss of privacy, the feeling of living in a glass box where every aspect of our existence is laid bare. Every hope, every fear, and every celebration feels shared, dissected, and documented before we can breathe it in as parents.

The hardest part is sharing Zoya. She is our daughter, our miracle, but in this environment, it feels like she belongs to everyone else. Decisions about her care are often out of our hands, and the protocols and processes of hospital life swallow up the moments that should be ours. There is no space to be a family, to hold her without someone watching, or to bond with her without someone interrupting.

The isolation within the NICU is unlike anything we have ever experienced. Yet, through it all, we stay for Zoya. We stay because she needs us, and we can't imagine being anywhere else while she fights to grow stronger. Every day, we tell ourselves that this is temporary, that one day, we will leave this place and reclaim the simple joys of being a family. The weight of living in this limbo leaves its mark, a deep, emotional ache that words can barely capture.

We endure so much alongside Zoya, sharing not just her struggles but the space around her with an entire hospital of people. It is exhausting, humbling, and isolating all at once. Yet, through it all, we hold onto the hope that one day, we will take her home, close the door behind us, and finally be her parents without the rest of the world looking in. That hope keeps us going, even on the most challenging days.

As we inch closer to the day Zoya finally comes home, that hope feels more tangible, more real. The long months in the hospital, each one stretching into the next, mold us into different versions of ourselves. We are no longer just parents but warriors, just like her. We face challenges we never could have imagined and battles we didn't know we were strong enough to endure. Yet, with every challenge and hardship, we realize we are not the same people we were months ago, we are stronger, more resilient, and more connected.

Zoya, our beautiful miracle, makes us believe in the impossible. Her fight becomes our fight, and her triumphs fuel our own. The road ahead remains uncertain, but we know we can handle whatever comes our way. Ultimately, it isn't the machines, the monitors, or the endless hospital protocols that get us through, it is our love for Zoya, a love so fierce and unbreakable that nothing can stand in our way.

The day we finally bring her home will not be a grand celebration with fanfare or a moment captured for everyone to see. It will be quiet, just the three of us, in the comfort of our own space. We will hold her, truly hold her, without the interruptions, the questions, or the endless rounds of medical professionals. We will be her parents in every sense of the word, fully, completely, without the gaze of the world upon us.

When the day of discharge finally comes, we will look back on this journey with gratitude. Grateful for the strength we discovered within ourselves. Grateful for the support we received from those who walked alongside us. Most of all, I am grateful for Zoya, who shows us what true courage looks like. Through her, we learn that there is always light, even in the darkest times. We are also deeply thankful for finding God along the way, for His guidance and strength throughout this journey, and for the blessings He has bestowed on our family in protecting and nurturing our sweet Zoya.

TRANSFER

This week is nothing short of eventful, filled with twists and turns that bring a rollercoaster of emotions. The news comes suddenly, catching us entirely off guard. Zoya's medical team informs us that she has made such incredible progress in her recovery that she is now stable enough to be transferred to the hospital nearest our home, Renown Regional Medical Center in Reno, Nevada. This revelation brings a rush of emotions, excitement, disbelief, and an underlying nervousness. For months, the NICU in Cleveland has been our world, and we've grown to trust the care and familiarity of her doctors and nurses. The idea of leaving that comfort behind for something unknown feels both thrilling and terrifying.

Until now, we've always imagined Zoya's discharge as a triumphant walk out of the hospital doors, with her snug in her car seat as we set off to start our life together. Yet, reality has a different plan. Her medical team explains that because Zoya still relies on oxygen support and an NG tube for feeding, there are significant challenges to consider, none more daunting than the 4,000-foot elevation change from

Cleveland to Reno. The higher altitude could put undue strain on her fragile respiratory system, making a commercial flight risky.

Their solution is a medical air transport staffed with professionals who can monitor her every second of the journey. It's a sobering reminder of how much care Zoya still requires, even in her stability. The decision to move her now is based on her excellent progress, the window of opportunity for insurance to approve such a costly and complex transfer is rapidly closing. If we wait too long, Zoya might no longer meet the criteria for coverage. Suddenly, we find ourselves in a whirlwind of preparations. We scramble to pack, wrap up loose ends in Cleveland, and prepare for what we think will be an imminent departure. The hospital staff told us we could leave within 24 to 48 hours. The idea of finally heading home to be closer to family and friends is exhilarating, but the speed of it all leaves us breathless.

As we brace for the move, reality hits, insurance approvals don't happen overnight. Days pass as we work with the hospital's discharge team, a fellow, and case managers to coordinate the transfer. Then, the news we dread arrives, the insurance denies the request.

We are devastated. The thought of being so close to this milestone, only to have it snatched away, is crushing. Yet, something doesn't sit right. We decide to take matters into our own hands and call the insurance company directly. What we uncover is almost too ridiculous to believe, the request has been sent to the wrong insurance company.

Fueled by frustration and determination, we make the necessary calls. First, we contact the correct insurance provider to confirm their process. Then, we reached out to Air Med International to have them resubmit the request, this time marked as urgent. It's the evening before the Thanksgiving holiday, and the air is charged with both urgency and chaos as we scramble to ensure all the paperwork is in order. With offices preparing to close and time slipping away, every second feels critical. Within an hour, we finally receive confirmation that the request is with the right people, a small but significant victory in the midst of the whirlwind.

Then comes the waiting. Every hour feels like an eternity. Finally, 48 hours later, the call comes, and Zoya's transfer is approved. Relief washes over us, followed by a new wave of emotions.

Excitement mixes with trepidation as we prepare for the journey ahead. We are leaving behind the team that has cared for Zoya since her very first days, the people who have fought alongside us through her toughest battles. The NICU in Cleveland has become a second home, and the idea of saying goodbye is bittersweet. Yet, the thought of being closer to home, closer to family, gives us hope and comfort.

As the transport date approaches, the logistics begin to take shape. Traveling on a Hawker 800 Jet with a specialized medical team that will oversee Zoya throughout the trip, monitoring her oxygen levels, heart rate, and overall condition. Thankfully, Trevor and I are cleared to accompany her on the flight to the new hospital in Reno. It isn't the picture-perfect homecoming we've envisioned, but it's another step closer to bringing her home for good.

As we prepare to fly Zoya to Renown in Reno, the air buzzes with anticipation. We've circled December 5th on the calendar. Everything has been meticulously planned, bags packed, goodbyes said, and our hearts set on this next step. Yet life, as it often does, throws us an unexpected curveball.

The news comes quietly but feels thunderous, the plane requires maintenance, and our departure is delayed. The deflation in the room is palpable. We've pinned so much hope on this day. Yet, amidst the disappointment, we resolve to refocus. December 7th becomes our new beacon of hope, and with unyielding determination, we turn our attention to preparing for this revised timeline. Friday arrives, bringing a mix of nervous energy and cautious optimism. We eagerly await the final clearance from Zoya's medical team and the receiving hospital in Reno. The moments tick by with agonizing slowness, but we believe the day's end will bring good news.

Instead, the knock on the door brings a tidal wave of devastation. The doctors enter, their faces a mix of sadness and concern. Reno's Renown Medical Center, our receiving hospital, informs our medical team that they no longer have room in their NICU to accommodate Zoya's transfer. Worse still, they have no plans to make space in the foreseeable future. The weight of those words is crushing. We've prepared ourselves for challenges, but this feels insurmountable.

Renown's NICU has never honestly planned to accept Zoya for an extended stay. Their intention, we discover, is a bait-and-switch, to accept her briefly before immediately transferring her to the Pediatric Intensive Care Unit (PICU).

Unlike the highly specialized and isolated NICU, where Zoya has spent her days surrounded by stringent precautions, the PICU is a different environment entirely, one that houses patients from 0 to 18 years old, many battling infectious diseases and viral illnesses. It's the last place our severely immunocompromised daughter should be.

For Zoya, this isn't just a logistical inconvenience. It's a matter of life and health. The very thought of exposing her fragile immune system to such a high-risk environment is unthinkable. The NICU in Cleveland has gone to extraordinary lengths to ensure her safety, isolating her from any potential exposure. The stark contrast to the PICU environment fills us with dread.

We are angry, heartbroken, and terrified. How can such a miscommunication and lack of preparation endanger Zoya's health? Our trust in this plan now feels shattered, replaced by a gnawing fear of the unknown.

Yet even in this storm of emotions, a glimmer of hope shines through. If there's one thing Zoya teaches us, it's that she is a fighter, and so are we. As her parents, we vow to continue advocating for her fiercely, navigating these challenges with the same tenacity that has brought her this far.

We also remind ourselves of a more profound truth. We believe it's God's plan for us to be here, and we trust that everything is as it should be. Though we may not fully understand the reasons now, we believe this journey is unfolding exactly as it is meant to. That faith carries us through the darkest moments and gives us hope for the brighter days ahead.

The journey to Reno may not unfold as planned, but it reflects the lengths we will go to ensure Zoya's safety and well-being. For her, we will always fight, adapt, and move forward, guided by love and trust in the path ahead. Though challenges remain, we are ready to face them together. Soon, Zoya will be closer than ever to the home that has been waiting for her all along.

TRANSPORT

After our first attempt to bring our sweet Zoya home falls through, we are heartbroken. Yet, as parents, there is no room for giving up. We know the challenges that lie ahead, and we persist. With every passing day, the window of opportunity to secure insurance approval for Zoya's care flight home grows smaller. An imminent yet ambiguous discharge day approaches, a milestone we eagerly want to celebrate, but it brings a daunting reality, getting Zoya home safely.

The alternative to a medical flight is unthinkable. Traveling on a commercial airline through three major airports, with layovers and crowded terminals, poses an enormous risk. Zoya's severely compromised immune system leaves her exceptionally vulnerable to infections. Each connection, each interaction, and each shared airspace with strangers represents a potential threat to her fragile health. This isn't just a theoretical concern, it is a life-and-health reality.

Zoya also faces the significant challenge of elevation changes. Our home in Reno, Nevada, sits 3,852 feet higher than her current location. For a baby with her medical history and delicate respiratory and cardiovascular systems, such a change could lead to complications like hypoxia. She needs medical professionals to monitor her closely and respond to any physiological changes. This is not a journey we can undertake without specialized care.

To make matters even more complicated, the NICU in Reno is at capacity. There are no alternative facilities that can accommodate her, leaving us with no other option but to ensure she can come directly home, not to another hospital, but home.

The fight for approval is nothing short of grueling. Although medical necessity is clear to us, convincing insurance providers requires relentless advocacy. We face roadblocks, setbacks, and moments of sheer frustration, yet we refuse to back down. This isn't just about transportation, it is about Zoya's life, safety, and future. After what feels like an uphill battle, we finally receive the news we have been praying for, approval for Zoya's care flight home.

We find out we are approved on December 20th, only five days before Christmas. We have been hoping and praying for a miracle to bring us home in time for the holidays. However, as we begin coordinating logistics, our hearts sink when we are told there are no available aircrafts, with scheduling likely to take more than a week. It is another race against the clock. If we don't get Zoya home before the new year, we must repay all our insurance deductibles, doubling our out-of-pocket costs. Desperation fuels us as we call and call, begging and pleading to get our sweet girl home.

My phone rings only a few hours later as Trevor and I eat lunch in the hospital cafeteria. Air Med International appears on the caller ID. My hands shake as I answer, and the flight coordinator asks if we can be ready to fly out tomorrow. I shout through tears of excitement, "Yes! Yes!" The moment feels surreal as they confirm the details and begin flight preparations. They inform us the aircraft will be a Learjet 35, a super small plane often compared to the equivalent of a sports car rather than a traditional aircraft.

Due to its size, only one parent can accompany Zoya on the flight. After much discussion, Trevor and I decide I will go with her. Knowing Trevor will have to wait until we land to hold her again is a bittersweet moment, but we both agree it is the best decision for our family.

Emotions run high as we prepare for the day, yet our guards are up. We are reluctant to fully embrace the approval, having been crushed so many times before. Each step toward the flight feels tentative, like holding our breath and bracing for the worst. Gratitude, relief, and a deep sense of accomplishment fill our hearts, but they mingle with caution. We think back to the months of uncertainty, the countless nights spent by her side in the NICU, the tears shed, and the prayers whispered. Now, we are one step closer to bringing her home, where she belongs.

We want to make sure Trevor gets home before us so he can be there waiting with open arms, ready to welcome his girls to our final home sweet home. After spending every waking second together for the last five months, it is scary to be apart. We are inseparable, my best friend, husband, and the best dad in the world. As we say our loving goodbyes, he kisses us both and heads for the airport at 3 a.m. on the morning of our care flight.

I can hardly fall back asleep after he leaves, so I focus on prepping, packing, and finalizing any last details. After so many doubts that the transport might fall through, it's finally real, Air Med International, along with a Physicians Ambulance Service team, arrives to transport our sweet girl to Burke Lakefront Airport. The care flight medical team runs all new leads to monitor her vitals and carefully places her onto a gurney. The sight of her tiny, resilient body on the full-sized gurney is overwhelming, the contrast is staggering. She looks so tiny, so fragile, yet so strong in the face of everything she has endured.

As the plane lifts off, tears stream down my face. This isn't just a flight but a lifeline, a bridge to the home we have longed for through endless days and nights in the NICU. The hum of the engines becomes a comforting rhythm, a constant reminder of our progress. Every mile feels like peeling away the layers of fear and uncertainty, replacing them with hope and anticipation. I sit beside her, watching her tiny chest rise and fall, marveling at her resilience, strength, and ability to inspire us never to give up. In those quiet moments in the sky, I whisper promises of the life waiting for her, of the love that will surround her every day.

The rush of emotions is overwhelming when the plane touches down in Reno. Zoya and I are transferred into our final transport home. They strap me onto the gurney and allow me to hold Zoya in my arms. Every bump of the gurney seems to echo the beating of my heart as if the journey we have just completed is finally settling within me. Pulling up to our home, the beacon of the ambulance lights flashes like a celebration of victory. The weight of everything we have endured feels lighter, almost surreal. The ambulance doors open, and there he is, Dad, standing proud, his eyes brimming with tears, arms outstretched. In that instant, the months of heartache, the sleepless nights, and the battles fought and won all seem worth it. As he holds us close, the world melts away, leaving only the warmth of his embrace and the realization that we have finally made it. Home. Not a word is spoken, but the love in that moment says everything.

Stepping through the door of our home feels like stepping into a dream. The sights and smells are familiar, yet everything feels new with Zoya in our arms. Her journey is nothing short of miraculous, and every detail of this day, the preparation, the flight, Trevor waiting for us, is a testament to the strength of family, the power of advocacy, and the determined spirit of one very special little girl. Zoya is home, she is safe, and she is exactly where she was always meant to be.

HOME

Bringing Zoya home is a dream that, for so long, felt like it was just out of reach. Now that we're here, the feeling is indescribable, a blend of overwhelming happiness, relief, and disbelief. It's almost as if the last five months existed in another lifetime, a parallel world where time moved differently. Those days in the hospital feel like a blur, as though they weren't real, yet every emotional detail is etched into our hearts, from the triumphs to the struggles. It was a surreal existence where we lived but didn't live, survived but didn't thrive.

Now, stepping out of that world and into our home feels like crossing a threshold into something we've yearned for with every fiber of our being. Carrying Zoya through the front door was a moment we had played out countless times in our minds, but the reality was even sweeter. To see her in her own space, in the room we carefully prepared for her, surrounded by the soft colors and tiny details we lovingly chose, feels like a blessing beyond measure.

Each moment at home reveals a new joy. The sterile, clinical environment of the NICU has been replaced with warmth, softness, and love. Instead of the persistent hum of monitors and the sterile beeps that once tracked her every heartbeat, we now hear the gentle rustle of her breaths as she sleeps, the quiet coos of contentment, and the soft melodies of lullabies filling the air. The quiet is no longer unsettling, it is a comfort.

The simple joys are the ones we treasure most. Holding her without wires tethering her tiny body, watching her stretch and yawn in the quiet of her own crib, or rocking her in the nursery as sunlight streams through the windows, each moment feels miraculous. Zoya's cries echo in the house, a sound that once might have been frightening but now feels like a song reminding us that she's here, she's home, and she's ours. Every smile, every coo, every tiny movement reminds us of how far she's come and how precious these moments truly are.

Even the most ordinary acts feel extraordinary as we marvel at the small luxuries we never knew we'd miss. Sitting together on the couch with Zoya nestled between us. Enjoying a meal at our dining table without having to leave the NICU because food wasn't allowed inside. Doing laundry in our washing machine instead of washing clothes in the sink and hanging them to dry for all to see. Sleeping in our own bed instead of curling up on a cold recliner chair and couch. Waking up to sunlight streaming through the windows instead of the fluorescent glare of the NICU. These simple comforts remind us how far we've come, making each day feel like a victory over the months we spent apart from this life.

Our journey to this point has been anything but ordinary. It's been filled with challenges, heartache, triumphs, and moments of grace. Zoya's strength and resilience have taught us more about love and perseverance than we ever thought possible. She is our miracle, our greatest blessing, and being home with her is everything we ever hoped for and more.

We still think about the NICU sometimes. Not because we miss it but because it's a part of our story. It's where Zoya proved her strength time and time again, where she showed us what it means to fight with grace and determination. As we settle into life at home, the NICU feels like a distant memory, a chapter we've finally closed.

Home is where Zoya belongs, where we belong. It's where we can finally exhale, shed the weight of the NICU, and step into the life we've dreamed of. Here, in the sanctuary of our own space, we begin to write a new chapter, one filled with hope, love, and the boundless joy of being a family at last.

We carry with us the lessons of the past five months: savor every moment, find joy in the smallest things, and never take the gift of family for granted. Home is no longer just a place, it's the feeling of being together, safe and whole.

BEGINNING

This is no ordinary ending but rather the beginning, the beginning of a beautiful life God has blessed us with. A life full of love, chance, and courage. Zoya's story is a testament to the strength we didn't know we had, the hope we dared to cling to, and the miracles that unfolded in the smallest, most unexpected ways.

To every parent who finds themselves in the dimly lit hallways of a NICU, surrounded by the beeping of monitors and the hum of ventilators, we see you. We know the weight of the questions you carry and the ache of the unknown. It is a world where time moves differently, measured not in hours but in heartbeats, progress, and the smallest victories. It is a place where you learn that courage isn't the absence of fear, but the resolve to love fiercely, to advocate boldly, and to celebrate every ounce gained and every milestone reached.

We remember the nights that stretched endlessly, the whispered prayers, and the desperate need to believe in a future that felt just out of reach. In those moments, we found grace. Grace in the strength of our tiny warrior, in the hands of the nurses who treated her as their own, and in the unwavering support of family and friends who held us up when we couldn't stand on our own. Every blood draw, every monitor alarm, every tear shed became part of a larger story, a story of love that refused to waver.

Zoya's journey taught us that life's greatest blessings often come wrapped in challenges. She showed us what it means to fight with every fiber of your being, to defy the odds, and to prove that love and faith can move mountains. Our hearts are filled with gratitude for the challenges we've overcome, the lessons learned, and the indescribable joy of knowing she is ours to cherish forever.

To the parents still in the thick of it, hold on. Hold on to the slivers of hope, the tiny victories, and the fierce love that keeps you going. Your journey will shape you in ways you can't yet imagine. It will teach you the depths of your resilience, the power of your voice, and the profound beauty of a single moment.

This story—Zoya's story—is a love letter to the parents who fight alongside their children, the medical teams who work tirelessly to save lives, and the babies who remind us of the strength that lies within even the smallest bodies. It reminds us that even on the darkest nights, light will find a way to shine through.

As we close this chapter, we step into a new one, not with fear but with boundless hope. As this is no ordinary ending. It is the beginning of a life brimming with promise, a life that will inspire others to believe in miracles and embrace the beauty of the journey, no matter how difficult it may seem.

To those walking this road, know that you are never alone. Your story matters, your child's story matters, and in the tapestry of life, every thread of struggle, triumph, and love weaves something breathtakingly beautiful.

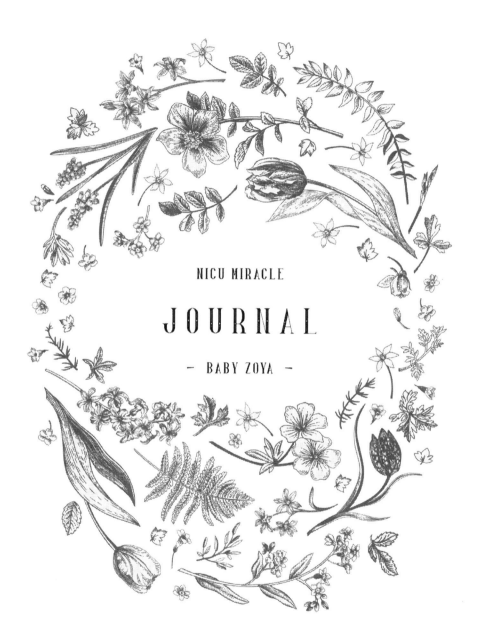

NICU MIRACLE

JOURNAL

— BABY ZOYA —

UPDATES

Day 3 | July 27, 2024

The best-case scenario continues, everything remains stable! Morning checkups and vitals are perfect with a strong heartbeat at 162 bpm. (The heartbeat range is 110-160 bpm; the higher the number, the happier and stronger she is)

Day 4 | July 28, 2024

Another perfect checkup! Her heartbeat is around 158 bpm, and she's been very active this morning, wiggling and kicking all around. We have an anatomy scan scheduled for Friday to see our little girl!

Day 5 | July 29, 2024

Baby Zoya is staying consistent with her strong heartbeat at around 150-160 bpm. We can't wait to see our little girl on Friday in the anatomy scan.

Day 6 | July 30, 2024

During our morning 20-minute fetal monitoring session, there were a couple of dips in her heartbeat. Protocol required us to stay on for an additional hour to gather enough data for review.

Our panel of doctors reassured us that this is completely normal for her gestational age. Everything still looks perfect, and the game plan remains unchanged!

Day 7 | July 31, 2024

All vitals and fetal monitoring went excellently this morning! Our baby girl is incredibly active; I can feel her wiggling and dancing from morning through night. She's even a little troublemaker, kicking the monitoring disk on my tummy while the doctors try to get her heartbeat!

Day 8 | August 1, 2024

Meet our perfect little girl, Zoya Pari Robinson, born on August 1st at 6:43 pm PST, weighing 1lb 8oz, measuring 11.42", gestational age of 23 weeks 5 days.

Our sweet baby girl is stronger than ever! She came into the world late last night, immediately crying and breathing on her own. She's so active and continues to move and wiggle, even responding to our touch by holding onto our fingertips.

Although strong and perfect we still have a long road ahead of us. She will remain in the MetroHealth NICU in Cleveland, OH for care until she is near full term or has the strength to be discharged from the hospital.

Baby Zoya is named after Lacey's great-grandmother, Zoja, who is considered our baby girl's guardian angel. It is a variant of the name Zoya, which has Greek roots and means "life." The name consistently signifies life and vitality. It is often associated with liveliness, energy, and a strong spirit.

Day 9 | August 2, 2024

Our baby girl is stronger than ever, breathing on her own, and still incredibly active. She's absolutely perfect! We're thrilled to be able to assist in her care, diaper changes, taking her temperature, and feeding her colostrum (milk) using tiny cotton swabs.

She has been incredibly stable, and while there may be challenges ahead, everything is looking very positive. We continue to see each and every second as a victory! From now on, we'll be providing weekly updates every Monday, sharing details about her care and growth.

Thank you all for the overwhelming love and support.

Day 12 | August 4, 2024

Our sweet baby girl is doing amazing. Yesterday morning, there were some quick changes to her care, including:

- Being put on an oscillator (a more dependent ventilator to help her CO_2 levels)
- Needing insulin (to help with glucose levels, which is normal and not related to being diabetic, the fluids she receives contain sugar, and when her fluids needed to be increased, she couldn't break down the sugar fast enough)
- Dopamine (to help blood pressure)
- A second dose of Curosurf (medicine to help the lungs)

Throughout the day, she handled all of these changes exceptionally well and was able to recover quickly. They've already drastically decreased her dependency on the oscillator, allowing her to breathe more independently, decreased her dopamine, and discontinued insulin.

Sleep has been light, but we managed to get a much-needed nap yesterday and are feeling good!

Zoya continues to amaze us with her strength, resilience, and recovery time! We are so proud of her!

DAY 13 | August 6, 2024

Little Princess is perfect today and is graduating off the oscillator! This means she will go back to entirely independent breathing, we're so proud of her!

DAY 19 | August 12, 2024

Sweet Zoya had an incredible week! She's 12 days old now, with a gestational age of 25 weeks. Her vitals are still strong, and last Wednesday, she was able to transition back to the conventional ventilator, meaning she's now breathing on her own with little assistance. The doctors are gradually weaning her off this ventilator and plan to remove her breathing tube as early as this week. After that, she'll switch to a noninvasive ventilator (NIV) with bi-nasal prongs.

Our little warrior also had both her umbilical catheters removed, which included her arterial catheter (UAC) and her parenteral nutrition (PN) line, previously used for blood sampling, blood pressure monitoring, and nutrition. To replace the umbilical lines, the doctors placed a peripherally inserted central catheter (PICC) line in a vein in her leg. This officially made our baby girl "wireless," and today, we get to hold her for the first time since her birth!

We're continuing to swab her mouth with breastmilk to help develop her digestive system. Plus, she's now officially receiving breastmilk as her main source of nutrition, delivered through a feeding tube, as she's still learning to coordinate swallowing and breathing at this age.

Last Friday, our little girl had her first poop! It might sound silly, but this is actually a big milestone. It's a key sign that her intestines are healthy and her digestive system is working properly. With her increased nutrition, she'll be plumping up in no time!

We couldn't be more proud of our little rockstar. Despite all the challenges she's faced, Zoya continues to amaze us with her strength and resilience. Every milestone she reaches fills our hearts with joy, and we're in awe of how far she's come. She's our little warrior, and we're so grateful to be on this journey with her, watching her grow stronger every day.

Measurement Monday:
Weight: 1lbs 7oz | Length: 12.6"
Head circumference: 8.27"
Arm circumference: 1.69"

Another fantastic week to share! Zoya is now 19 days old with a gestational age of 26 weeks, and she's doing incredibly well. Her vitals are strong, and she's started a new weekly medication called Darbepoetin, which helps her produce red blood cells and reduces the need for blood transfusions. This is really exciting because we want to limit transfusions as much as possible. So far, she's only needed one, which the doctors say is amazing for her gestational age. Zoya is part of a NICU program called Minimal Donor Exposure, where she's matched with a single blood donor and will stay with that same donor for any future transfusions.

Last Tuesday, she was extubated, which means she transitioned to a noninvasive ventilator (NIV) with bi-nasal prongs. She's breathing on her own, with just a little assistance to keep her lungs from fully deflating and to help them stay open during exhales. By Wednesday, there was a small amount of fluid in her lungs, raising some concerns about her heart known as Patent Ductus Arteriosus (PDA). This is a completely normal and expected occurrence in all babies, where a small blood vessel in the heart that usually closes after birth remains open. It's more common in preemies since it can take a bit longer to close compared to full-term babies, where it usually closes within 24 hours after birth. PDA can affect blood flow between the heart and lungs, but thankfully, Zoya had a cardiac ultrasound (Echo) and was cleared! The doctors say her heart is strong, with no issues detected, and her heart development is looking great!

In other exciting news, we got to hold our little warrior princess for the first time this week! The moment she was placed on my chest was the most emotional and profound experience of our lives. As we held her close, tears filled my eyes as I mentally captured our perfect little family of three for the very first time. The moment was magical.

Zoya's umbilical cord fell off this week, revealing the most adorable little belly button we've ever seen! It feels like such a big milestone, and we couldn't be more thrilled to see this sweet little detail emerge.

Another exciting moment happened when our little girl opened her eyes! We've been eagerly waiting for this, and it was so special to finally see her bright, curious eyes taking in the world around her. It's amazing to think about all the new sights she'll be experiencing as she continues to grow. Each day, she's showing us more of her personality, and these moments are truly unforgettable.

Measurement Monday:
Weight: 1lbs 7oz | Length: 12.6"
Head circumference: 8.5"
Arm circumference: 1.77"

DAY 33 | August 26, 2024

Zoya is now 26 days old, with a gestational age of 27 weeks. Things have been going wonderfully for our baby girl over this past week. Her vitals have stayed strong with minimal changes, and she's been able to increase her milk intake, which is helping her gradually wean off the Total Parenteral Nutrition (TPN). TPN delivers nutrients directly into her bloodstream, bypassing the digestive system. The nutrients include sugars, amino acids (protein), vitamins, minerals, electrolytes, and lipids (fats). It's been a very strong and consistent week for her, which is the best-case scenario for maintaining her stability.

It's been a month since we were admitted to MetroHealth Hospital in Cleveland, and it's starting to feel like home. We couldn't imagine being anywhere else than right by her side. The plan remains the same, she'll stay here until she's close to full term or strong enough to be discharged and go home. We're hoping that will be around November 23rd, her original due date. We're so proud of our little princess!

Measurement Monday:
Weight: 1lbs 10oz | Length: 13"
Head circumference: 8.75"
Arm circumference: 1.57"

DAY 39 | September 2, 2024

It's been 39 days since I was originally admitted to the ER here in Cleveland, and now Zoya is 33 days old, having celebrated her 1-month milestone on the 1st, with a gestational age of 28 weeks.

Zoya faced a tough week due to anemia and an infection. Things escalated quickly early Wednesday morning after her 2 a.m. care when her vitals became increasingly unstable. Her CO_2 levels were high, her blood count was low, and her white blood cell count was elevated, indicating an infection.

They immediately started her on antibiotics and sent her blood for a culture. The culture results were more of a formality, as they were already covering all potential infections with the current medication.

Zoya has remained very active, moving her arms around, which might seem like a small thing, but the doctor mentioned that her alertness and movement are positive signs. It shows that she's not completely exhausted by whatever she's fighting off, which is encouraging.

The following morning, she received her second blood transfusion, which marked a significant turning point in her recovery. The transfusion greatly helped improve oxygen delivery, stabilized her vital signs, and prevented complications like apnea and bradycardia. It also boosted her immune system and overall stability.

Over the remaining week, she's been closely monitored and has shown an incredibly resilient recovery. All her vital signs and blood work have vastly improved, and she's a very alert and happy girl! Things are definitely on the mend. Our princess is so tough!

Measurement Monday:
Weight: 1lbs 14oz | Length: 13.46"
Head circumference: 9.05"
Arm circumference: 2.46"

DAY 46 | September 9, 2024

Sweet Zoya is now 6 weeks old, with a gestational age of 29 weeks, and she's growing so much and is doing wonderfully! She made a strong recovery from her infection and is off all antibiotics. Last Thursday, she received her third blood transfusion, which further improved her oxygen delivery, stabilized her vital signs, and boosted her immune system and overall stability.

This past week marked a major milestone, we started practicing breastfeeding! Even though the coordination of sucking, swallowing, and breathing usually develops around 34-35 weeks, Zoya has shown early signs of being ready. It was a big moment when the doctors decided to let her give it a try, and she did an amazing job, impressing her entire care team! Right now, she's using a "non-nutritive latch," which means she latches and sucks without actually drawing out any milk. This stage is all about getting her familiar with the process and practicing for when she's ready to coordinate all three actions together. For now, all her nutrition still comes from her TPN and nasogastric (NG) tube, as she's still too premature to be fed orally. When the time comes, we'll be ready!

Measurement Monday:
Weight: 2lbs 4oz | Length: 13.62"
Head circumference: 9.64"
Arm circumference: 2.26"

DAY 53 | September 16, 2024

This has been our toughest week yet, as we've received some challenging news on Wednesday about Zoya's health. She has been diagnosed with two severe conditions: Necrotizing Enterocolitis (NEC) and a Cytomegalovirus (CMV) infection. NEC is a serious intestinal disease that primarily affects premature babies, causing inflammation and potentially leading to the destruction or death of bowel tissue. An initial X-ray showed minor developments of NEC, where abnormal gas patterns were visible in the walls of her intestines, giving them a bubbly appearance. The CMV infection further complicated her situation, weakening her immune system and contributing to a significant drop in her platelet levels, which required four platelet transfusions and another blood transfusion to stabilize her. Thankfully, both conditions were caught extremely early, allowing the medical team to intervene quickly.

On top of everything else, Zoya had an eye exam on Friday, since premature infants are at high risk for a condition called retinopathy of prematurity (ROP). ROP occurs when the blood vessels in a baby's eyes develop abnormally, potentially leading to vision problems or, in severe cases, retinal detachment, which can result in blindness if not treated. The risk of developing ROP is particularly high in babies born before 31 weeks of gestation or with a very low birth weight. Thankfully, we received some much-needed good news from the pediatric ophthalmologist: her eyes are developing perfectly for her gestational age, and there are no concerns at this time. Although her eyes are currently only 40-50% developed, they will continue monitoring her every two weeks to ensure her eyes are progressing properly. The good news is that ROP is treatable, and so far, everything looks promising.

Remarkably, within just 48 hours, Zoya made an incredibly strong recovery, with her symptoms improving so rapidly that her doctors are not only amazed but are now questioning if the diagnosis of NEC might have been incorrect. Her symptoms resolved so quickly that they wonder if it may be solely the CMV infection at play, as both conditions can cause a drop in platelets. However, to ensure all bases are covered, they plan to continue treating her as if she still has both conditions. Zoya is now happy, alert, active, and showing that feisty spirit we know and love, giving us even more hope as we move forward. Your thoughts and prayers mean the world to us and our little warrior.

Measurement Monday:
Weight: 2lbs 10oz | Length: 14"
Head circumference: 9.8"
Arm circumference: 2.6"

DAY 60 | September 23, 2024

We're happy to report that Zoya has had a positive week of recovery! At 7 weeks old now, with a gestational age of 31 weeks, she continues to show us just how strong she is.

There's not much to report this week as we're still focused on the tail end of her recovery from last week. However, everything is progressing smoothly, and we're thrilled with the direction she's headed. Zoya remains her joyful, high-spirited self, constantly amazing us with her strength and resilience.

We're incredibly grateful for the progress she's made and look forward to more good news in the coming weeks.

Measurement Monday:
Weight: 3lbs 2oz | Length: 14.6"
Head circumference: 10.25"
Arm circumference: 2.75"

DAY 67 | September 30, 2024

It's now been 67 days since I was first admitted to the ER here in Cleveland, and Zoya will soon be celebrating her 2-month milestone on October 1st, with a gestational age of 32 weeks.

Zoya continues to battle a few challenges as her recent conditions haven't completely resolved. In addition to her regular care team, she has a network of pediatric experts in Endocrinology, Nephrology, and Infectious Diseases. These specialists have been consulted to ensure that nothing serious, like syndromes or diseases, are being missed. Fortunately, everything points to her issues being related to the prematurity of her organs and immune system, which brings some relief to everyone.

Right now, the focus is on balancing her electrolytes, with the primary concern being her phosphorus levels. Zoya is struggling to retain phosphorus, as her body is flushing it out through urine faster than expected. Phosphorus is crucial for the development of healthy bones and teeth, as well as for proper muscle and nerve function. Since she's still so young, keeping her phosphorus levels stable is vital for her growth and overall development.

The medical team is closely monitoring this and continually adjusting her treatment to help her body retain the phosphorus it needs. They're hopeful that with these adjustments, her levels will stabilize soon, and they remain confident that she'll continue making progress.

Measurement Monday:
Weight: 3lbs 12oz | Length: 15"

Head circumference: 10.62"
Arm circumference: 3.14"

DAY 74 | October 07, 2024

Zoya is now 9 weeks old with a gestational age of 33 weeks, and our brave little girl has faced another challenging week. She's been struggling to retain some of her micronutrients, which has led to the need for 24-hour supplement infusions and daily bloodwork to monitor her levels. Unfortunately, the increased frequency of blood draws required another blood transfusion. Zoya has endured nearly 20 IV attempts this week, many of them unsuccessful, and just yesterday, her last accessible vein failed. As a result, we've had to switch to adding the supplements to her breast milk feeds.

However, adding supplements to her feeds isn't necessarily bad news. As Zoya continues to grow and her feed amounts increase, she's able to receive more nutrition through her milk rather than relying on her TPN via her PICC line. This is a positive step forward in her development, as it means her body is getting stronger and better equipped to process nutrients through natural feeding.

There are so many exciting milestones coming up for Zoya as she grows stronger and becomes more stable. Here's what we are looking forward to in the coming weeks:

Transitioning out of her temperature-controlled isolette and into a crib! This will be a big step in her development and independence as she learns to regulate her body temperature on her own.

Reducing her nasal INV support and progressing to CPAP, with the eventual goal of moving to Vapotherm. Each reduction in respiratory support is a huge achievement and shows her lungs are getting stronger.

Breastfeeding! As Zoya's feeds increase and she becomes more stable, we are looking forward to starting the process of breastfeeding.

Each of these milestones represents the key criteria the hospital uses to gauge Zoya's progress and assess her readiness for independence from the NICU, bringing her closer to discharge. She needs to regulate her temperature, breathe on her own, and feed independently. We are eagerly looking forward to celebrating each achievement as she continues to grow and thrive.

Measurement Monday:
Weight: 4lbs 6oz | Length: 15.31"

Head circumference: 10.83"
Arm circumference: 3.15"

Day 81 | October 14, 2024

Saturday marked a special milestone, at 34 weeks gestation, I would have been induced to deliver baby Zoya. The goal being, that she remained in my tummy after my Prelabor Rupture of Membranes (PPROM), which is the medical way of saying my water broke at just 22 weeks. Reflecting on the past 10 weeks of her beautiful existence, I can't help but feel how blessed we are to have gained all this extra time with her, as I wouldn't have even met her until now.

She had a wonderful week and is getting stronger and more stable with each passing day. We are hoping she'll hit a couple big milestones this week, and we can't wait to share our update with you next Monday!

Measurement Monday:
Weight: 5lbs 0oz | Length: 16.14"
Head circumference: 11.02"
Arm circumference: 3.15"

Day 88 | October 21, 2024

Zoya is 11 weeks old, with a gestational age of 35 weeks.

Late last night, unexpectedly, a surgeon was called to do a small procedure on her hand. She had developed an abscess, and an infection called cellulitis, which needed immediate attention. The operation went very quickly, and our little girl was so brave throughout the entire process. Though it was a nerve-wracking moment, we're relieved that she is already responding well to the treatment, and her medical team is closely monitoring her recovery. A specialized hand surgeon will also be reviewing her X-ray and ultrasound imaging to determine if any further treatment is necessary.

Today, she has a follow-up exam with her pediatric ophthalmologic surgeon to monitor a condition called retinopathy of prematurity (ROP). We're hopeful that her eyes will continue to develop properly, as she is at high risk for this condition. The encouraging news is that ROP is treatable, so regardless of the outcome, we're staying optimistic.

Other than the most recent news, our big girl had a fantastic week, reaching a major milestone last Wednesday, she's now off Total Parenteral Nutrition (TPN)! Her IV nutrition through the PICC line is complete, allowing for its removal, bringing her closer to being fully wireless. Now, her only nutrition comes from breast milk and supplements through her nasogastric (NG) tube.

Zoya has also made significant progress with her breathing treatments and is now on Vapotherm, one of the last devices she needs to wean from. The next goal is to gradually reduce her airflow support, as the current level is too high for safe oral feeding and could lead to aspiration. Once the airflow is lower, the final steps will be to feed independently, and then we can finally come home!

As exciting as all of this is, it looks like we're still in for another month or so, likely extending beyond her original due date of November 23rd.

Measurement Monday:
Weight: 5lbs 0oz | Length: 16.5"
Head circumference: 11.4"
Arm circumference: 3.2"

Day 95 | October 28, 2024

Our sweet Zoya is 12 weeks old and has been stable enough to move out of her isolette and into a crib! This has been an incredibly emotional and exciting milestone for us. Seeing her in a crib has felt like such a significant step toward normalcy, a hopeful sign that our strong little girl is growing and progressing. Moving to a crib symbolizes a little victory, a glimpse of

her someday being in her own crib at home. We are so proud of her resilience, knowing how much she fought to get to this point.

Measurement Monday:
Weight: 4lbs 15oz | Length: 16.6"
Head circumference: 11.6"
Arm circumference: 3.2"

Day 102 | November 04, 2024

Zoya is now 13 weeks old, with a gestational age of 37 weeks. Moving her to a crib recently seems to have sparked a new phase in her growth. This week, she's made incredible progress, her airflow support was drastically decreased, and today she tried bottle feeding for the first time. Watching her take that bottle was a heartwarming moment and a huge step forward.

Another big achievement this week has been the stability of her lab results. Seeing her numbers stay consistent is a major milestone, showing just how hard Zoya is working to keep her vitals steady. Every day, she's getting stronger, and we're so proud of her determination. Each of these little victories brings her one step closer to coming home.

Zoya also got to celebrate her very first Halloween, dressed up as a "prisoner of the NICU"! Her costume was a hit with the staff, who couldn't stop smiling and laughing at her little outfit. One of her doctors even went above and beyond, knitting a tiny ball-and-chain to complete the look. It was a sweet, funny moment that brought some much-needed lightness and joy to everyone around her.

Measurement Monday:
Weight: 5lbs 8oz | Length: 16.9"
Head circumference: 11.8"
Arm circumference: 3.2"

Day 109 | November 11, 2024

Zoya is 14 weeks old, 102 days to be exact, with a gestational age of 38 weeks. She's been making remarkable progress every day in her development. Last Wednesday, she took a bottle for the very first time, impressing everyone with how well she's handling it. She began slowly, starting with a 5ml bottle, then moved up to 10ml by Thursday, 15ml on Friday, 25ml on Saturday, and is now taking an impressive 30ml by bottle!

Her next milestone is to consistently complete her full PO feeds of 45ml by mouth for 48 hours, which would mean her NG tube can be removed! ("PO" stands for "per os," a Latin term for "by mouth," referring to oral feeding). Her care team is so proud of her bottle-feeding skills, especially since it can be a challenge for preemies to master the coordination of sucking, swallowing, and breathing.

We're so excited to see what the next few weeks hold for Zoya's progress and can't wait to share more updates. For the first time, I can truly feel the light at the end of the tunnel, and the dream of bringing her home feels closer than ever.

Measurement Monday:
Weight: 6lbs 1oz | Length: 17.4"
Head circumference: 12.1"
Arm circumference: 3.4"

Day 116 | November 18, 2024

This week is an extra special one for our family. On Saturday, we mark Zoya's original due date, November 23, 2024. It's incredible to reflect on her journey over these past 15 weeks. At 39 weeks gestation, Zoya has grown stronger and more resilient each day, and we are so proud of her progress.

There isn't much new to report this week, which is a blessing in itself. Zoya continues to do well on her PO feeds and oxygen, steadily moving in the right direction. She's stable and thriving, which gives us so much peace and hope as we look toward the future.

She still has a bit more growing to do before she's ready to come home, but every milestone she reaches reminds us just how far she's come since those early, uncertain NICU days. Her strength and determination inspire us daily, and we're looking forward to what the next few weeks will bring as we inch closer to finally bringing her home.

Measurement Monday:
Weight: 6lbs 11oz | Length: 17.8"
Head circumference: 12.5"
Arm circumference: 3.4"

Day 123 | November 25, 2024

Zoya is officially considered a full-term baby at 40 weeks gestation, celebrating her original due date of November 23, 2024. Reaching this moment is deeply emotional for us. It feels like we've waited a lifetime for this day to arrive, and now that it's here, we are overwhelmed with gratitude and joy. The thought that we would only just be meeting her now is truly mind-blowing. Instead, we've been blessed with nearly four full months of bonding with her, caring for her, and witnessing her blossom. These precious months have allowed us to see her tiny personality emerge, each moment a gift that has filled our hearts with more love than we ever imagined possible.

This is also the week of Thanksgiving, and we couldn't be more thankful for our family and the progress our sweet girl has made. While our celebration looks a little different this year, just me, Trevor, Zoya, and a box of pizza, it's definitely one to remember. This simple gathering, filled with love and hope, reminds us that even in the most unexpected circumstances, there is so much to be thankful for.

Zoya continues to do well, and her stability has been a blessing. She's thriving on her feeds and oxygen, and she amazes us every day with her strength and determination.

Zoya continues to do well, and her stability has been a blessing. She's thriving on her feeds and oxygen, and she amazes us every day with her strength and determination.

Measurement Monday:
Weight: 7lbs 4oz | Length: 18.11"
Head circumference: 12.6"
Arm circumference: 3.5"

Day 130 | December 02, 2024

Zoya is 4 months old while being just one week old, corrected age. There have been some recent changes in her progress, and her medical team has determined that she is stable enough to be transferred to a hospital in Reno. A transfer had never been discussed before, and this decision was made quickly. Her team explained that the window to qualify for insurance coverage of medical transport was closing, requiring us to make a firm decision within 24 to 48 hours. Zoya still relies on oxygen, and an NG feeding tube, and the most concerning factor is the elevation change from Cleveland to Reno, a difference of approximately 4,000 feet. This raised significant concerns about her ability to adjust, and her team felt that a care flight would be the safest way to get her home.

This situation has been overwhelming to process, requiring us to manage the logistics of packing, traveling, and ensuring everything is in place for Zoya's care at the new facility. Beyond the practicalities, we've had to face the emotional reality of leaving behind what has been our home for the past four months. Questions about what "home" will look like, how our lives will adjust, and trusting a new medical team with our precious daughter's care have weighed heavily on our hearts. The emotional weight of this transition has been profound.

Above all, we're ready to continue her journey in Reno, one step closer to bringing her home for good

Measurement Monday:
Weight: 7lbs 9oz | Length: 18.3"
Head circumference: 12.8"
Arm circumference: 3.6"

Day 137 | December 09, 2024

Zoya is 4 months old, while being just two weeks old, corrected age. We're thrilled to share some incredible milestones Zoya has reached this week! Her NG tube has been removed, and she's been taking all her PO feeds by mouth like a champ. Watching her make such strides in feeding has been such a joy and a huge relief.

In addition, her oxygen needs have been steadily decreasing. She's gone from 3/4 to 2/4 to 1/4, and now she's down to an eighth. These are such promising steps toward being fully independent of oxygen support.

We are so proud of Zoya and the progress she's making every single day. Thank you all for your continued prayers, love, and support as we celebrate these wins. Your encouragement means the world to us.

Measurement Monday:
Weight: 8lbs 1oz | Length: 18.8"
Head circumference: 13.4"
Arm circumference: 3.9"

Day 144 | December 16, 2024

Zoya is 4 months old, while just three weeks old, corrected age. Her oxygen progress continues to improve, and she has officially weaned to the final stage of just 0.8 L of oxygen. We even got to try her on room air, which was a moment we will never forget.

For the first time in nearly 5 months, we saw her beautiful face without her nasal cannula and all the tape. Seeing her sensitive red cheeks finally free of constant tape was so emotional, it felt like seeing her in a whole new way. Zoya did absolutely incredible during her trial and managed an impressive 3.5 hours without any support at all!

While she wasn't quite ready to breathe completely on her own just yet, this was such a huge step. She's back on minimal oxygen support now, and this will help her prepare for traveling home soon, especially to ensure she can handle the increased elevation.

Measurement Monday:
Weight: 8lbs 9oz | Length: 19.1"
Head circumference: 13.6"
Arm circumference: 4"

Day 151 | December 23, 2024

We are thrilled to share some wonderful news this week, Zoya has officially made it home! After months of dedicated care in the NICU and the incredible work of her medical team, Zoya was safely care-flighted back to Reno and is now settling in at home with us.

This moment feels like a dream come true. Bringing her home is a huge milestone, and we couldn't have done it without all of the love, prayers, and support from each of you along the way.

Zoya has adjusted beautifully so far. We're enjoying the simple joys of having her with us, her coos, her stretches, and just being able to hold her in the comfort of our home. It's been such a heartwarming and emotional time.

We're taking it one day at a time, cherishing these moments, and creating new memories as a family. Thank you again for being part of Zoya's journey, it means the world to us!

PRAYERS

Dear God, Please watch over little Zoya, keep her safe and strong each day. Help her feel all the love around her, and let her smile in every way. Give her strength and give her courage, as she grows and as she plays. Thank you for our special Zoya, we love her more than words can say. Amen.

— Mom & Dad

Lacey and Trevor, Though Zoya was early, we know in our hearts that she will be okay. When we came to see her, we know that she is getting the best care. Being a part of her first days of life is something we cherish, and can't wait to see her again soon. We keep praying for her strength to develop and grow into the precious baby girl that she deserves to be. She is truly a miracle. We love you all with all our hearts!

— Grandma & Grandpa

Hi sissy I love you and I'm praying for you, and Zoya I am so glad parents and Trevor are there with you. Good night sissy love you so much!

— Cassi S.

Zoya, Lacey, and Trevor, With all our prayers and the hundreds praying for Zoya and family, we know the Miracle Baby will continue to grow and be one great young lady. All our Love Grandma and I for all of you.

— Great Grandma & Grandpa

I can't imagine how you guys are feeling. But I do know God works miracles and he has a beautiful plan for Zoya. Me and the girls will be praying every day for strength and growth for Zoya, and you. And for all the doctors and nurses to have healing hands and wisdom to know just what she needs. I know this will be a long journey with a lot of unknown but God will be there through it all. I can't wait to meet Zoya and give you a big hug! We all love you guys so much.

— Missy M.

Welcome to Baby Girl Zoya! She looks so strong. I'm thinking of you all and I hope you're doing ok.

— Kaitlyn R.

So happy you and Zoya are doing ok. I'm not a godly man but I've been praying almost every day to whoever would listen for both your health. I know it's still a long journey ahead but I am relieved everything is going well so far. Love you all and can't wait to meet the newest member of the family!

— Troy C.

Hey Lace. I was thinking about ya. Jayme filled me in a few days ago. Just wanted to say hi and that I hope all is well. We're praying for you both to be able to come home soon! I am so happy to hear she's doing well and growing stronger! We are thinking of you all and love you guys!! I'm sorry you had to go through such a scary thing! Much love to you, Trevor, and baby Zoya.

— Michael M.

I can't even imagine how you're all feeling. I am so happy to hear you guys are okay and I'm confident it will continue that way. She's a strong girl like her momma and I know you guys will make it out of this stronger than ever. I love you so much and will be thinking about you every single day so please keep me posted. I wish you were here so I could visit you. My heart is with you.

— Shelby M.

I'm thinking positively and praying so hard for you and baby Zoya. You're strong and I love you so much, I'm always here for you. I wish I could hug you, I am so proud of you and Zoya's strength. Love you both so much. Beautiful princess Zoya Auntie Carly loves you so much!

— Carly D.

We are thinking of you nonstop throughout these moments you are strong and resilient and so is your sweet baby girl she will grow up hearing of her miraculous journey here and her strength and her momma's strength from day one, sending you guys all the love in our hearts.

— Alyssa D.

I just wanted to reach out to make sure you're ok. We love you and are praying for both of you. I've had a few family members with similar situations because all my sister's kids were preemies. They all turned out fine. I believe you both will be fine as well.

— Meng H.

Hi Babygirl! Just wanted to let you know I was thinking about you and you are in my prayers. I love you.

— Maureen L.

My friend, let me know if I can help you with anything, really! Our prayers are for you and your beautiful little baby! Everything will be okay! The Focus right now is on your baby, nothing else matters! That's really the mindset you should have! If you really have to stay living over there, I'm sure you'll be okay along with a beautiful a healthy baby! We are keeping our prayers stronger than ever over here. Soon enough, this whole thing will be behind you, and you'll be enjoying your baby at home, safe and sound!

— Gabriel A.

I hope you are doing okay, I haven't experienced this but I know it is scary. I wish you both strength and love. I know I'm far but if there is anything I can do please reach out. Also, I do believe congratulations are in order you are a mom with a beautiful girl already wearing a signature bow.

— Shante M.

Hi babes, I am sending all the love and positive energy your way. I love you and baby Zoya very much. If there is anything I can do for you, please let me know!

— Rachael O.

Omg my whole heart, she's going to grow up to be so beautiful and strong thank you for keeping me updated I'm excited to see her grow healthier each and every day I love you so much!!!

— Payton R.

Hey you! I didn't want to bug you, I talked to Jayme and he told me what's been going on and I just wanted to say we are all thinking of you! Please let us know if there's anything we can do!

— Tony Jr. Evans

You, Trevor, and baby Zoya are in our family's prayers. First of the month! Strong baby girl!!! Fighter! Thinking of you.

— Shelby S.

I am so sorry for all that has happened. I literally just heard the news. My heart aches for you. Please let me know if there is anything at all I can do.

— Justin H.

You're holding your baby! I'm praying time passes quickly as she continues to thrive and grow and you're on your way home.

— Lenny Sue T.

Just checking in to see how our beautiful mommy-to-be is doing I know this has been quite a stressful situation for you, but certainly, you are in all of our prayers !!! If there's anything we can do for you certainly don't hesitate to ask! Looking forward to the arrival of beautiful baby ZOYA !!!

We are all happy to help and we know that God is going to bless you with a gorgeous, sweet, creative, talented baby girl who will be very healthy. I know how frightening this whole situation has been and rightfully so I would feel exactly the same as you do! The good news is, though you will rise above, and things will work out. Just let us know whatever we can do to help. I can tell that you're a very direct person so just be direct and give us our marching orders. We are here in our team Lacey and team ZOYA!!!

I was praying for you at church yesterday. There was a special statue of the Virgin Mary mother of God touring and I lit a candle for you all and said some prayers for good things good health happiness and love always!! How fortunate is she to feel so loved by mommy daddy family and friends God bless her and God bless both of you for having such patience through this whole situation.

—   Jeannie G.

A P G A R   S C O R E

Our baby girl's first report card…

The APGAR score is a rapid assessment of a newborn's health conducted at one, five, and ten minutes after birth.

APGAR Score | One Minute After Birth

Score Legend:

< 7 - May need help. **4 to 6** - Needs assistance breathing. < 3 - Needs immediate help.

Apgar Sign	0	1	2
A Activity (muscle tone)	☐ None, limp, or muscles are floppy	☐ Some flexion of arms and legs	☒ Active motion and flexion; arms and legs resist extension
P Pulse (heart rate)	☐ Absent or no heart rate	☐ Less than 100 beats per minute	☒ At least 100 beats per minute
G Grimace (reflexes)	☐ No response to stimulation	☒ Facial grimace during stimulation or suction	☐ Cries, pulls away, coughs, or sneezes upon stimulation
A Appearance	☐ Body is blue or pale	☒ Pink body with bluish extremities (hands/feet)	☐ Body and extremities are pink
R Respiration (breathing)	☐ Not breathing	☒ Weak, slow, or irregular breathing	☐ Strong crying; normal rate of breathing

Total score: 7/10

APGAR Score | Five Minutes After Birth

Scoring Legend: < 6 - Needs more medical help.

Apgar Sign	0	1	2
A Activity (muscle tone)	☐ None, limp, or muscles are floppy	☐ Some flexion of arms and legs	☒ Active motion and flexion; arms and legs resist extension
P Pulse (heart rate)	☐ Absent or no heart rate	☐ Less than 100 beats per minute	☒ At least 100 beats per minute
G Grimace (reflexes)	☐ No response to stimulation	☐ Facial grimace during stimulation or suction	☒ Cries, pulls away, coughs, or sneezes upon stimulation
A Appearance	☐ Body is blue or pale	☒ Pink body with bluish extremities (hands/feet)	☐ Body and extremities are pink
R Respiration (breathing)	☐ Not breathing	☐ Weak, slow, or irregular breathing	☒ Strong crying; normal rate of breathing

Total score: 9/10

HEIRLOOM

This cross, rich in history and meaning, is a cherished family heirloom passed down through generations. Originally belonging to my great-grandmother Zoja Pari, who was born in 1909 has survived the trials of time and war, carrying with it the weight of our family's journey. Zoja's father, Minister Rajevski of the Eastern Orthodox Church, christened her with this crucifix as a symbol of faith and protection. She wore it as she fled Estonia during WWII, burying all other valuables, keeping only this cross.

This traditional Eastern Orthodox crucifix, though worn smooth and faded by time, holds profound and enduring meaning. The Estonian inscription on the back, "päästa ja kaitsta" ("save and protect"), is a timeless prayer, reflecting the faith and hope carried through generations. The markings above Christ on the front symbolize the sacred "INRI" (Jesus of Nazareth, King of the Jews). Once adorned with the "IC XC" inscription for "Jesus Christ" on the left and right sides of the cross, it also featured a skull at the base of the crucifix, representing Christ's victory over death, a powerful reminder of faith's enduring strength through hardship. Now smoothed by the passage of time, the crucifix reflects the countless hands and heartfelt prayers that have held it over generations.

This cherished heirloom, passed from Zoja to my grandmother, to me, and soon to you, baby Zoya, is a profound symbol of faith, love, and resilience. It carries with it a legacy of protection and strength, guiding each generation it touches. More than a representation of faith, this cross stands as a testament to resilience, having been safeguarded during my great-grandmother's escape from Estonia, a country ravaged by war. Hidden, protected, and preserved amidst great adversity, its journey reflects the enduring importance of family heritage and the unbreakable bond that connects us across generations.

When I was admitted to the hospital with you, baby Zoya, your great-grandma Viive gave me this cross, and I clung to it with all my heart. It has become more than just a necklace to me, it has become my source of strength, my constant reminder of the love and protection that has always surrounded our family. As I pray each day, I whisper words of hope and healing not only to God but to your great-great-grandmother Zoja, and to all of the angels who watch over you. I ask for their guidance and blessing on you, as you begin your journey into this world. With each prayer, I feel a sense of peace wash over me, trusting that the same strength that protected my family will protect you.

Sweet Zoya, this cross will soon be yours. As I place it in your hands, I want you to know that it carries with it not just the stories of our family but the love, protection, and strength that has been passed down through every generation. This is not just a necklace, it is a symbol of everything we hold dear: the love that binds us, the faith that sustains us, and the courage that helps us overcome. Just like your namesake, Zoya, you carry within you a legacy of incredible strength, courage, and grace. Already, in your first few months, you have shown your own remarkable strength during your time in the NICU, proving to be a fighter with a spirit as fierce as the women who came before you.

May this cross remind you that no matter where life takes you, you are never alone. You are always surrounded by the love of your family, the wisdom of their stories, and the grace of God. This cross is a piece of us, just as you are, my darling Zoya. You are the next generation in a beautiful story, one filled with love, faith, and the enduring power of hope. May it always remind you of how deeply you are loved.

LETTERS

My Sweet Zoya,

As I sit here, gazing at your tiny but incredible presence, just 1 pound, 8 ounces of pure miracle, my heart is overflowing with emotions that words can't fully capture. Playing back every moment of your existence, and as I write this letter, I am writing the story of you. A story of strength, courage, and love that began long before you arrived and continues to unfold with every breath you take.

You are our precious little miracle, and even though you're so small, you've already made a world-sized impact on our lives. In your own way, you have touched the world around you, sparking love, hope, and strength in so many hearts.

I want to thank you. Thank you for choosing us to be your parents, for showing us what true courage and resilience look like, and for giving us the greatest gift we've ever received, the gift of being your mom and dad. You are, without a doubt, the greatest happiness we've ever known. Your father and I have never experienced a joy this pure and complete. Every day with you is a blessing, and we feel honored to be your parents.

I want to love you. I love you more than words will ever express, more than the stars love the night sky, and more than the ocean loves the shore. My love for you is infinite, boundless, and grows stronger with every breath you take. It fills every beat of my heart, every thought in my mind, and I will always, always be there for you, guiding, protecting, and surrounding you with love. You are part of me, in every way, my heart living outside of me.

I want to pray for you. I pray every day that you continue to grow strong, healthy, and safe. With each passing moment, you will develop and thrive in ways that remind us of the miracle you truly are. I pray that the world will always be kind to you, that you will never lack love, and that you will be surrounded by people who cherish you as much as we do. I pray for your health, your happiness, and your future.

I want to cherish you. Every moment with you is a treasure I hold close. Every tiny movement, every breath, every blink is something I never take for granted. I will cherish every milestone, every laugh, every tear, every joy, and even every challenge we may face together. You are a gift, and I will always hold you in my heart, never taking for granted the miracle that you are.

I want to teach you. There are so many things I want to share with you as you grow. I want to show you how to be brave, how to stay curious, and how to keep learning, and most importantly, the love of family. I want to show you the beauty in the world, the strength within yourself, and the power of your own spirit. I want to guide you, support you, and watch you grow into the amazing person I know you will become.

But most of all, I want to bring you home. I dream every day of the moment we can walk out of these doors together and take you to the place where you truly belong. Where your room is waiting, where we can finally begin our life as a family in the way we've always imagined. Your home is with us, and we can't wait to show you the love, warmth, and joy that fills it.

Until that day comes, we are here with you, every step, every breath, every heartbeat. We believe in you, sweet Zoya. You've already proven to us and the world how strong you are, and we know you will continue to amaze us in ways we can't even imagine.

With all my love, forever and always,

Mom

My Dearest Trevor,

When I think back on everything we've endured these past five months, my heart overflows with gratitude, love, and admiration for you. You've been my anchor through the most challenging time of our lives, and I can't imagine how I would have made it through without you.

From the moment I was admitted to the hospital, everything about our journey changed. In those vulnerable moments, confined to a hospital bed and consumed by fear, you became my protector, my advocate, my safe haven, and my home.

This journey has tested us in ways we never could have imagined. There were moments when I wasn't sure how we'd keep going, but you always found a way to remind me that we're a team and that together, we can face anything. Even on the hardest days, you gave me the strength to keep going. Time and time again, you've shown me why you are not just my husband but my best friend and greatest blessing.

You've given me the most precious gift of all, a family. You've made my dream of becoming a mother come true, and together, we've brought our beautiful baby girl into this world. Zoya is our miracle, a reflection of everything we've built together: our love, our strength, and our hope.

Watching Zoya fight in the NICU has been both the hardest and most beautiful experience of my life. You've poured every ounce of your heart into loving and supporting her, and I know she feels it. Every time I see you hold her tiny hand or look at her with so much love, my heart swells. The way you love, care for, and fight for her is everything I ever dreamed of in a husband and father. She's so lucky to have you as her dad.

You've shown Zoya what it means to have a father who will always fight for her, who will always be there no matter how hard the road ahead might seem. You've shown me what it means to have a husband whose devotion is unwavering, even under the heaviest burdens.

When I look at Zoya, I see a future brighter than I ever imagined. I see your care and tenderness reflected in her eyes and the strength and resilience she's inherited from you. She's our joy and greatest achievement, and none of it would have been possible without you.

You've given me so much, you've given me strength when I had none, hope when I felt lost, and above all, a family. Watching you as a father has been one of the greatest privileges of my life. Through this journey, I've fallen even more deeply in love with you, and I know I'll keep falling for the rest of my life.

One day, when Zoya is older, we'll tell her about all of this. We'll share the story of her time in the NICU, the challenges we faced, and the love that carried us through. I can't wait to tell her about her incredible dad, a man who never wavered, who loved her fiercely from the start, and who has been my rock through it all.

Thank you for being the man you are. Thank you for loving me, for loving Zoya, and for making sure I never felt alone, even in the hardest moments. I love you more than words can ever express, and I always will.

With all my love, forever and always,

Lacey